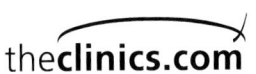

VETERINARY CLINICS OF NORTH AMERICA

Equine Practice

Trauma and Emergency Care

GUEST EDITOR
Eileen K. Sullivan, DVM, MS

April 2007 • Volume 23 • Number 1

SAUNDERS

An Imprint of Elsevier, Inc.
PHILADELPHIA   LONDON   TORONTO   MONTREAL   SYDNEY   TOKYO

W.B. SAUNDERS COMPANY
A Division of Elsevier Inc.

Elsevier, Inc., 1600 John F. Kennedy Blvd., Suite 1800, Philadelphia, PA 19103-2899

http://www.vetequine.theclinics.com

VETERINARY CLINICS OF NORTH AMERICA:
EQUINE PRACTICE
April 2007
Editor: John Vassallo; j.vassallo@elsevier.com

Volume 23, Number 1
ISSN 0749-0739
ISBN-13: 978-1-4160-4378-2
ISBN-10: 1-4160-4378-0

Copyright © 2007 by Elsevier Inc. All rights reserved. No part of this publication may be reproduced or transmitted in any form or by any means, electronic or mechanical, including photocopy, recording, or any information retrieval system, without written permission from the Publisher.

Single photocopies of single articles may be made for personal use as allowed by national copyright laws. Permission of the publisher and payment of a fee is required for all other photocopying, including multiple or systematic copying, copying for advertising or promotional purposes, resale, and all forms of document delivery. Special rates are available for educational institutions that wish to make photocopies for non-profit educational classroom use. Permissions may be sought directly from Elsevier's Rights Department in Philadelphia, PA, USA: phone: (+1) 215 239 3804, fax: (+1) 215 239 3805, e-mail: healthpermissions@elsevier.com. Requests may also be completed on-line via the Elsevier homepage (http://www.elsevier.com/locate/permissions). In the USA, users may clear permissions and make payments through the Copyright Clearance Center, Inc., 222 Rosewood Drive, Danvers, MA 01923, USA; phone: (978) 750-8400, fax: (978) 750-4744, and in the UK through the Copyright Licensing Agency Rapid Clearance Service (CLARCS), 90 Tottenham Court Road, London WIP 0LP, UK; phone: (+44) 171 436 5931; fax: (+44) 171 436 3986. Other countries may have a local reprographic rights agency for payments.

The ideas and opinions expressed in *Veterinary Clinics of North America: Equine Practice* do not necessarily reflect those of the Publisher. The Publisher does not assume any responsibility for any injury and/or damage to persons or property arising out of or related to any use of the material contained in this periodical. The reader is advised to check the appropriate medical literature and the product information currently provided by the manufacturer of each drug to be administered to verify the dosage, the method and duration of administration, or contraindications. It is the responsibility of the treating physician or other health care professional, relying on independent experience and knowledge of the patient, to determine drug dosages and the best treatment for the patient. Mention of any product in this issue should not be construed as endorsement by the contributors, editors, or the Publisher of the product or manufacturers' claims.

Veterinary Clinics of North America: Equine Practice (ISSN 0749-0739) is published in April, August, and December by Elsevier Inc., 360 Park Avenue South, New York, NY 10010-1710. Business and Editorial Offices: 1600 John F. Kennedy Blvd., Suite 1800, Philadelphia, PA 19103-2899. Customer Service office: 6277 Sea Harbor Drive, Orlando, FL 32887-4800. Subscription prices are $165.00 per year for US individuals, $265.00 per year for US institutions, $83.00 per year for US students and residents, $193.00 per year for Canadian individuals, $324.00 per year for Canadian institutions, $209.00 per year for international individuals, $324.00 per year for international institutions and $105.00 per year for Canadian and foreign students/residents. To receive student/resident rate, orders must be accompanied by name of affiliated institution, date of term, and the *signature* of program/residency coordinator on institution letterhead. Orders will be billed at individual rate until proof of status is received. Foreign air speed delivery is included in all *Clinics* subscription prices. All prices are subject to change without notice. **POSTMASTER:** Send address changes to *Veterinary Clinics of North America: Equine Practice*, Elsevier Periodicals Customer Service, 6277 Sea Harbor Drive, Orlando, FL 32887-4800, USA; phone: 1-800-654-2452 [toll free number for US customers], or 1-407-345-4000 [customers outside US]; fax: 1-407-363-1354; e-mail: usjcs@elsevier.com

Reprints. For copies of 100 or more, of articles in this publication, please contact the Commercial Reprints Department, Elsevier Inc., 360 Park Avenue South, New York, New York 10010-1710. Tel. (212) 633-3813, Fax: (212) 462-1935 email: reprints@elsevier.com.

Veterinary Clinics of North America: Equine Practice is covered in *Index Medicus, Excerpta Medica, Current Contents/Agriculture, Biology and Environmental Sciences,* and *ISI*.

Printed in the United States of America.

TRAUMA AND EMERGENCY CARE

GUEST EDITOR

EILEEN K. SULLIVAN, DVM, MS, Diplomate, American College of Veterinary Surgeons; Assistant Professor of Equine Surgery and Critical Care, Department of Clinical Sciences, College of Veterinary and Biomedical Sciences, Colorado State University, Fort Collins, Colorado

CONTRIBUTORS

LAWRENCE R. BRAMLAGE, DVM, MS, Diplomate, American College of Veterinary Surgeons; Partner, Rood & Riddle Equine Hospital, Lexington, Kentucky

BARBARA DALLAP SCHAER, VMD, Diplomate, American College of Veterinary Surgeons; Diplomate, American College of Veterinary Emergency and Critical Care; Assistant Professor, Department of Clinical Studies, George D. Widener Hospital for Large Animals, University of Pennsylvania School of Veterinary Medicine, New Bolton Center, Kennett Square, Pennsylvania

DIANA M. HASSEL, DVM, PhD, Diplomate, American College of Veterinary Surgeons; Assistant Professor, Equine Emergency Surgery and Critical Care, Colorado State University, Fort Collins, Colorado

JOLYNN JOYCE, DVM, Resident, Equine Lameness and Surgery, Department of Clinical Sciences, Colorado State University, Fort Collins, Colorado

GABRIELE A. LANDOLT, DVM, PhD, Diplomate, American College of Veterinary Internal Medicine; Assistant Professor of Equine Medicine, Department of Clinical Sciences, College of Veterinary Medicine and Biomedical Sciences, Colorado State University, Fort Collins, Colorado

PEGGY S. MARSH, DVM, Diplomate, American College of Veterinary Internal Medicine; Diplomate, American College of Veterinary Emergency and Critical Care; Clinical Assistant Professor, Department of Large Animal Clinical Sciences, College of Veterinary Medicine, Texas A&M University, College Station, Texas

REBECCA S. McCONNICO, DVM, PhD, Diplomate, American College of Veterinary Internal Medicine; Associate Professor of Equine Medicine, Equine Health Studies Program, Department of Veterinary Clinical Sciences, Louisiana State University School of Veterinary Medicine; Equine Branch Director, Louisiana State Animal Response Team, Baton Rouge, Louisiana

MARGARET C. MUDGE, VMD, Assistant Professor of Equine Emergency and Critical Care, Department of Clinical Sciences, The Ohio State University, School of Veterinary Medicine, Columbus, Ohio

JONATHAN E. PALMER, VMD, Diplomate, American College of Veterinary Internal Medicine, Associate Professor of Medicine, Section of Large Animal Medicine; Section of Anesthesia, Emergency and Critical Care Medicine, School of Veterinary Medicine, University of Pennsylvania; Chief, Neonatal Intensive Care Service, Director of Perinatal/Neonatal Programs, Graham French Neonatal Section, Connelly Intensive Care Unit, New Bolton Center, University of Pennsylvania, Kennett Square, Pennsylvania

CARL SOFFLER, DVM, Resident, Equine Internal Medicine, Department of Clinical Sciences, Colorado State University, College of Veterinary and Biomedical Sciences, Fort Collins, Colorado

BRETT S. TENNENT-BROWN, BVSc, Diplomate, American College of Veterinary Internal Medicine; Fellow in Emergency and Critical Care, Department of Clinical Studies, University of Pennsylvania School of Veterinary Medicine, New Bolton Center, Kennett Square, Pennsylvania

TRAUMA AND EMERGENCY CARE

CONTENTS

Preface xi
Eileen K. Sullivan

Flood Injury in Horses 1
Rebecca S. McConnico

> There is no way to prepare for every situation that arises in a disaster. By working closely with other producers and agricultural leaders, however, horse owners can lessen the impact of a disaster on their operation. Preparation and detailed planning are the most important aspects of flood-related injury prevention. Encouraging animal owners and caretakers to have an evacuation plan and dispersing knowledge about local and regional disaster authorities are critical for a successful disaster response. Educational programs on future disaster response empower communities to care for their people and animals responsibly.

Fire and Smoke Inhalation Injury in Horses 19
Peggy S. Marsh

> Although not common in horses, fire and smoke inhalation trauma may require veterinary assistance at several levels. Most commonly, the equine clinician is called on to provide care of potentially complex and emotionally charged cases. Thermal injury, along with smoke inhalation, can cause local and diffuse lesions. Massive tissue edema may occur, which can be a challenge to manage as well as creating organ dysfunction at distant sites. Further complications of severely affected patients are varied and include life-threatening sepsis. This article reviews some of the important features of this type of trauma.

Management of Equine Poisoning and Envenomation 31
Gabriele A. Landolt

Acute poisoning and envenomation often represent a diagnostic and therapeutic challenge. Although identification ultimately may benefit the affected animal, treatment frequently must commence before an etiologic diagnosis is established. Therefore, the goals for the management of acutely intoxicated horses must be focused on emergency intervention and stabilization of the patient, prevention of further exposure, and aggressive decontamination. This article reviews the treatment steps that should be considered during the management of horses experiencing poisoning or envenomation.

Ophthalmic Emergencies in Horses 49
Barbara Dallap Schaer

The emergency clinician is frequently in the position of receiving, evaluating, and initiating treatment on horses with ophthalmic emergencies or orbital trauma. In the best of circumstances, an ophthalmologist is available to guide initial therapy and ultimately assume responsibility for the management of the patient during the remainder of its hospitalization, but this is not always the case. The information presented here is meant to provide the emergency clinician with basic guidelines for the initial assessment and management of horses sustaining ocular injuries or presented with an ophthalmic emergency. The article provides initial information regarding prognosis, descriptions of indicated diagnostics and procedures that may need to be performed on an emergency basis, and suggestions regarding early therapy. Whenever possible, the management of such cases should be overseen or assumed by a veterinary ophthalmologist after the emergent stabilization of the patient.

Thoracic Trauma in Horses 67
Diana M. Hassel

Thoracic trauma represents an important cause of morbidity in mortality after injury in human beings and animals. After any form of suspected chest wall trauma, initial emergency management should include assurance of a patent airway and adequate ventilation, along with treatment for shock if present. As with any open wound, tetanus prophylaxis should be instituted. Types of trauma to the thoracic region of the horse include pectoral and axillary lacerations, penetrating chest wounds, flail chest, fractures of the ribs, blunt thoracic trauma, and several potential sequelae that include pneumothorax, pneumomediastinum, hemothorax, pleuritis, fistulae of the sternum or ribs, and diaphragmatic hernia. Emergency management of these various forms of thoracic trauma is discussed.

Trauma with Neurologic Sequelae 81
Brett S. Tennent-Brown

Spinal cord injury (SCI) in horses may arise from rearing and falling backward, collisions, kicks, and slipping. The pathophysiology of SCI comprises a primary mechanical injury followed by a cascade of secondary events. These secondary events include microvascular ischemia, oxidative stress, excitotoxicity, ion dysregulation, and inflammation. It is often the severity of secondary injury that limits the restoration of neurologic function. Clinical signs after SCI depend on the location of the lesion and the relative amount of damage to the gray and white matter. Acute management of SCI should include optimization of oxygen delivery to the injured tissues. A brief discussion of some of the more promising medical therapies that have been investigated in human medicine and may be applicable to equine patients is included.

Injury to Synovial Structures 103
JoLynn Joyce

Injuries to synovial structures are common in horses and may be life threatening or career ending if severe. Early recognition and initiation of aggressive treatment in the form of appropriate systemic and local antimicrobial therapy and surgical treatment improve the likelihood of a good outcome. Chronic injuries and delayed treatment may result in progression of infection into tendons, bone, and other structures, thus complicating treatment and resulting in a poorer prognosis for return to function.

Field Fracture Management 117
Margaret C. Mudge and Lawrence R. Bramlage

Emergency management of distal limb and skull fractures in horses is vital to the successful outcome of these cases. Distal limb fractures, in particular, require careful assessment and counseling of the owner as well as adequate stabilization or coaptation of the fracture. Horses with limb or skull fractures may also have concurrent pain, blood loss, and other fluid losses that can result in shock requiring fluid therapy before definitive treatment of the fracture. Proper emergency fracture stabilization, initial treatment in the field, and patient transport are discussed.

Oxidative Stress 135
Carl Soffler

Oxidative stress refers to the cellular injury and pathologic change that occurs when there is an imbalance favoring oxidants over antioxidants within a living organism. In human medicine, oxidative stress has been implicated in numerous disease processes, which has led to further research into the clinical benefits and efficacy of antioxidant therapy. The evaluation of oxidative stress in the horse has been limited primarily to ischemia-reperfusion injury of the gastrointestinal tract, recurrent airway obstruction, exercise, osteoarthritis, equine motor neuron disease, and pituitary pars intermedia dysfunction. Each of these is examined in this review in terms of the current evidence for oxidative stress as well as the evidence for current antioxidant therapy in equine medicine and the potential of future research and therapies. Oxidative stress research is currently an emerging field with relevance to the equine critical patient.

Neonatal Foal Resuscitation 159
Jonathan E. Palmer

Cardiac arrest in foals is generally secondary to other serious systemic diseases. Although it can often be anticipated, a clear plan is vital to success. Establishing cardiac output through chest compressions is the most important first step. This step should be followed by ventilation, drug therapy, identifying the nonperfusing cardiac rhythm, and following a preplanned treatment algorithm. Birth resuscitation requires special treatment considerations. The clinician should be prepared to perform resuscitation any time a birth is attended.

Index 183

FORTHCOMING ISSUES

August 2007
    Evidence-Based Veterinary Medicine
    David Ramey, DVM, *Guest Editor*

December 2007
    Urinary Tract Disorders
    Harold C. Schott II, DVM, PhD, *Guest Editor*

April 2008
    Orthopedic Challenges in Performance Horses
    Antonio Cruz, DVM, MVM, MSc,
    Guest Editor

RECENT ISSUES

December 2006
    Advances in Reproduction
    Elaine M. Carnevale, DVM, PhD,
    Guest Editor

August 2006
    Advances in Diagnosis and Management of Infection
    Louise L. Southwood, BVSc, PhD,
    Guest Editor

April 2006
    Medical Case Management
    Jennifer M. MacLeay, DVM, PhD, *Guest Editor*

The Clinics are now available online!

Access your subscription at:
www.theclinics.com

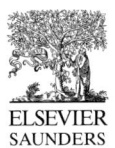

Preface

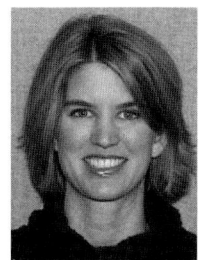

Eileen K. Sullivan, DVM, MS
Guest Editor

It has been my privilege to serve as Guest Editor for this issue of *Veterinary Clinics of North America: Equine Practice* focusing on trauma and emergency care. The authors were selected to address issues of importance in specialized areas of emergency medicine. This issue offers a "one-resource" approach to trauma, the first of its kind. Readers are directed to the flood injury section, wherein coordination of a veterinary response to massive flooding is outlined. Aspects of fire injury are summarized, and included is systematic documentation of burn victims. Other modes of injury, such as poisonings and oxidation, are covered in depth. Penetrating and blunt traumas are grouped by anatomic location and organs affected to allow for direct reference. Finally, on-farm foal triage is explained with practical methods.

Special thanks are due to Dr. A. Simon Turner, Consulting Editor, for the opportunity to be involved in this project, and to John Vassallo at Elsevier/Saunders for his support and guidance. Special thanks are also extended to an entire generation of veterinarians who develop reflex tachycardia in response to a telephone ring and whose repertoire does not include phrases such as "Thank goodness, it's Friday"—progress in emergency medicine is a direct result of your efforts.

Eileen K. Sullivan, DVM, MS
Department of Clinical Sciences
College of Veterinary and Biomedical Sciences
Colorado State University
300 West Drake Road
Fort Collins, CO 80523, USA

E-mail address: eileen.sullivan@colostate.edu

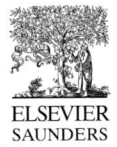

VETERINARY
CLINICS
Equine Practice

Flood Injury in Horses

Rebecca S. McConnico, DVM, PhD[a,b],*

[a]Equine Health Studies Program, Department of Veterinary Clinical Sciences, Louisiana State University School of Veterinary Medicine, Skip Bertman Drive, Baton Rouge, LA 70803, USA
[b]Louisianna State Animal Response Team, Baton Rouge, LA, USA

Floods are the most common weather-related disasters known on earth and occur throughout the United States, causing billions of dollars in damage and threatening the lives of people and animals. The average yearly financial loss attributable to floods in the United States averages $6 billion [1]. Flooding damages infrastructure and depresses economic activity [1]. Flood-related livestock injuries and death make up a major component of these losses, affecting the economic and emotional welfare of livestock producers, including horse owners.

The principal causes of floods in the eastern United States are hurricanes and storms. In the western United States, causes include snowmelt and rainstorms. The Midwest flooding in 1993 and damage caused by Hurricanes Katrina and Rita in 2005 are the three costliest flood events in US history, estimated at $20 billion and more than $60 billion, respectively. The United States Geological Survey (USGS) mapping of flood-prone areas of the United States is extensive (Fig. 1), with greater than 85% of the United States having had at least one disaster declaration related to a flooding situation.

Planning and prevention

Horse owners must be proactive in taking responsibility for protection of the animals under their care. Advanced planning can help horse owners to minimize the loss of animal lives and the health problems associated with disasters, such as floods. Because of the vulnerability of coastal regions to

---

* Equine Health Studies Program, Department of Veterinary Clinical Sciences, Louisiana State University School of Veterinary Medicine, Skip Bertman Drive, Baton Rouge, LA 70803.
 E-mail address: mcconnico@vetmed.lsu.edu

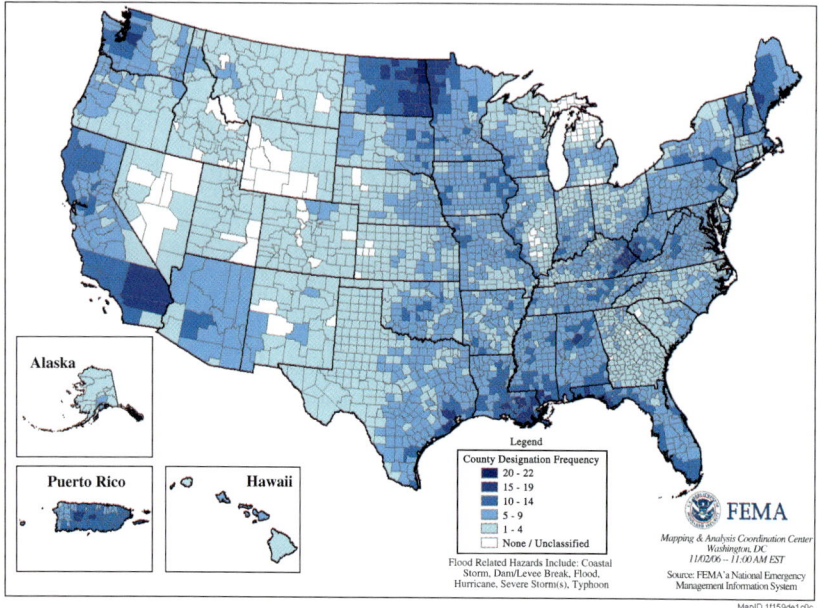

Fig. 1. Flood map (2006). Presidential disaster declarations related to flooding in the United States, 1964 through 2006, are shown by county or Louisianna parish. (*Courtesy of* Federal Emergency Management Administration [FEMA], Washington, DC.)

hurricanes and storms and the potential widespread damage caused by flooding, preparedness in these most vulnerable areas is essential. It must be stressed that although help may be available from many sources after a disaster, owners themselves are ultimately responsible for the welfare of their animals and should prepare accordingly. Well in advance of a potential disaster situation, horse owners and producers should evaluate their herd health programs with their veterinarian. Horses that undergo evacuation related to disaster response are stressed and are likely to commingle with other horses and livestock. Herd biosecurity is breeched, which makes increasing herd immunity imperative. Pneumonia and abortions should be anticipated and can be minimized with proper herd nutrition and vaccination. Before storm seasons, horses should be vaccinated with current strains for equine herpesvirus 1 and 4 and equine influenza 1 and 2 in addition to the encephalitides (eastern equine encephalomyelitis [EEE], western equine encephalomyelitis [WEE], and West Nile virus [WNV]) and tetanus.

Animal identification is critical. If horses are evacuated and commingled or escape and are later captured, it is essential to be able to identify the herd of origin. Many horses look alike; thus, permanent brands, lip tattoos, or electronic identification that is unique to each animal or to each farm or ranch is essential. The US Horse Industry Equine Species Working Group advisors to the US Department of Agriculture (USDA) National Animal Identification System recommends electronic microchip identification using International Standards Organization/American National Standards Institute (ISO/ANSI)-compatible radiofrequency identification (RFID 117.84/ 85, 134.2 kHz) as the standard equine identification method to ensure uniformity and compatibility [2]. A single microchip should be implanted deep in the horse's nuchal ligament midway between the poll and the withers on the left side. Photographs or videotapes of horses may also help in the identification process. Horses should have two forms of identification: a permanent form (microchip, lip tattoo, or brand) and a visible tag or marking with the owner's name and current contact information. Livestock paint sticks, etching using an electric clipper with a no. 40 blade, a permanent marking pen, and bright spray paint are household products that can be used to identify horses (Fig. 2). Official guidelines for predisaster visible identification of horses are not available, but current recommendations are to include, at a minimum, the owner's name and current viable contact telephone number or e-mail address. Copies of herd records, proof of ownership, and registration papers should be stored in a safe and secure location.

In situations like an impending hurricane, where advanced warning may be given, health papers should be provided by a veterinarian if horses are to be evacuated, particularly if there is a possibility of the horse traveling across state lines. In case of events in which widespread evacuation is recommended, including that of horses (eg, category 3 or greater hurricanes), state or federal veterinary officials are the authority for determining travel requirements necessary for interstate transport of evacuated livestock. Official health papers or an official Coggin's test result (proof of negative equine immunodeficiency anemia status) may suffice. In some situations, it may not be possible to evacuate or rescue all animals. Owners may need to prioritize so that their most valuable animals receive attention first.

Because of the possibility of mass evacuation of many animals, plans should be made weeks in advance of a potential disaster. Owners should partner with other farms and ranches to provide transportation and evacuation space so that public holding areas can be used for rescued animals. Biosecurity issues should be discussed when making these arrangements. Producers should have safe efficient handling facilities ready in advance. Livestock trailers should be inspected to make sure they are ready for hauling long distances. If flooding or high winds are expected and animals cannot be evacuated, they should be left in large open pastures and not placed in barns. Unable to flee or escape their confines during the flooding after Hurricane Katrina, hundreds of horses drowned because owners left them locked in their stalls thinking they would be safe from flying debris (Fig. 3). Horses that were able to make it to high ground survived (Fig. 4).

State animal response teams (SARTs) are taking the lead in many states in coordinating animal disaster preparedness efforts [3–5]. Owners

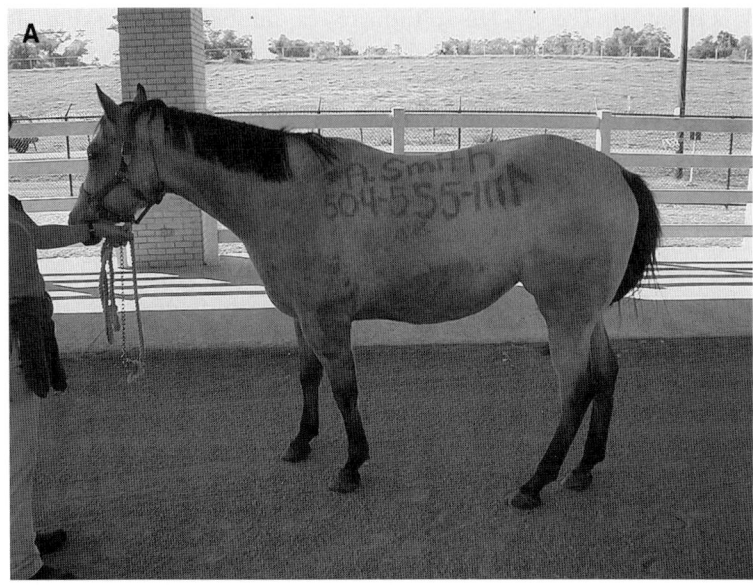

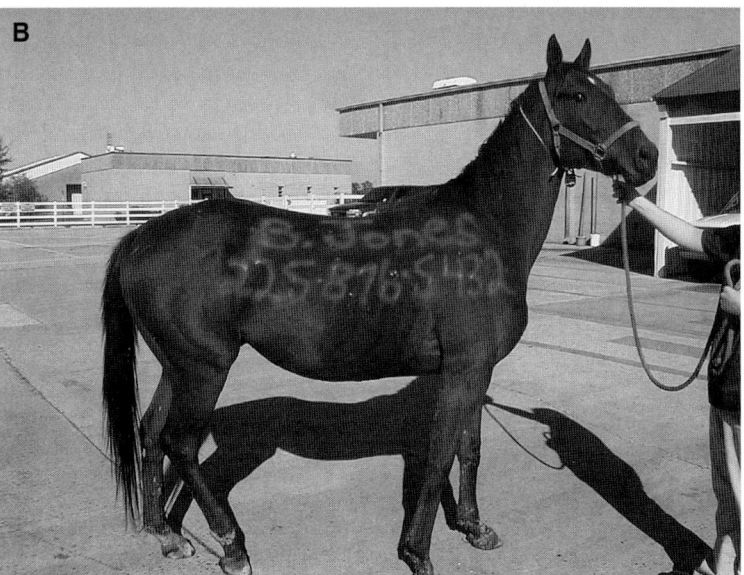

Fig. 2. Predisaster body marking with horse owner name and contact information using livestock paint stick (*A*) and fluorescent spray paint (*B*). (*Courtesy of* Rebecca McConnico, DVM, PhD, Baton Rouge, LA.)

should take an active part in coordinating and making known their plans with these organizations and other local lead agriculture-related groups, such as agriculture extension agencies; the USDA's natural resource conservation services and farm service agencies; local farm bureaus; state,

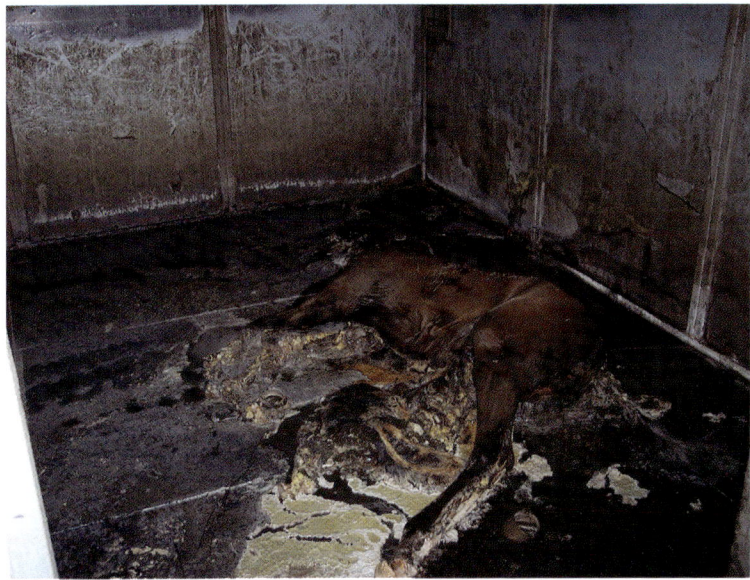

Fig. 3. Weanling horse left in the stall during Hurricane Katrina. Note the hoof marks and water line on the stall walls where the horse attempted to escape. (*Courtesy of* Leslie Talley, Baton Rouge, LA.)

regional, or local producer groups; livestock auction markets; and feed stores. Different tasks, such as livestock hauling; feed, fuel, and generator acquisition and distribution; and animal evacuation, rescue, and treatment, should be assigned to individuals or groups in advance. Primary and contingent holding areas for evacuated or rescued livestock (eg, show facilities, race tracks) as well as staging areas for feed and fuel distribution should be identified in advance. Special evacuation routes for livestock should be considered so that loaded trucks and trailers can keep moving to avoid development of heat stress in transported animals. Along with the numerous human lives lost during the traffic gridlock evacuation of the Texas and Louisiana coastal regions before the landfall of Hurricane Rita (autumn of 2005), hundreds of horses and cattle perished because of heat stress while being transported. Roads may be closed to trailer and towing traffic as a storm approaches. Early evacuation is imperative to avoid these problems.

In large-scale disasters involving large numbers of livestock, providing food and fresh water to animals that have been sheltered or pastured in-place, is the first priority. Owners should have enough emergency hay and water sources for 3 to 5 days, because most rescue and response efforts go toward saving human lives first. Adult horses need 5 to 15 gal of water per head per day. Storage tanks previously holding chemicals should not be used to store water. If wells depend on electricity to pump water, hand

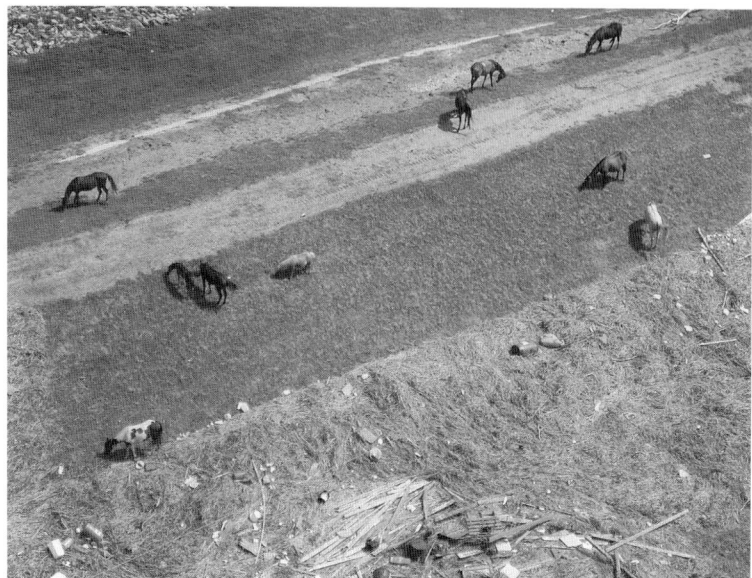

Fig. 4. Horses able to escape to high ground (levees) survived the storm surge and flooding in Plaquemines Parish, Lousiana, in September 2005 during the aftermath of Hurricane Katrina. Note the debris fields on either side of the levee. (*Courtesy of* Leslie Talley, Baton Rouge, LA.)

pumps or generators should be available in case of electrical outages. Producers should make their local extension office aware in advance of the numbers of animals and their locations. This helps to ensure that your animals are included in immediate feed distributions if available. Otherwise, feed may not be distributed until this information can be verified, which puts the animals at risk.

Response

In flood situations, horse owners are often frantic and demanding. It is important for communities to have a livestock plan that includes trained personnel and resources so that reasonable decisions can be made quickly to save lives as well as to meet the urgent health-related needs of flood-affected horse victims. Horse owners should do their part to evacuate ahead of a flood and to make sure that their horses can be haltered and handled. For example, in the aftermath of Tropical Storm Allison (2001 in Louisiana), a horse farm owner located near the Red River overflow area in central Louisiana requested rescue and evacuation of 16 horses because his farm land and barn would soon be flooded [6]. On arrival, veterinarian and animal technician rescue crews found that more than half of these horses were not wearing halters and that they were not congregated in a safe paddock holding area. The horses were difficult to gather and restrain,

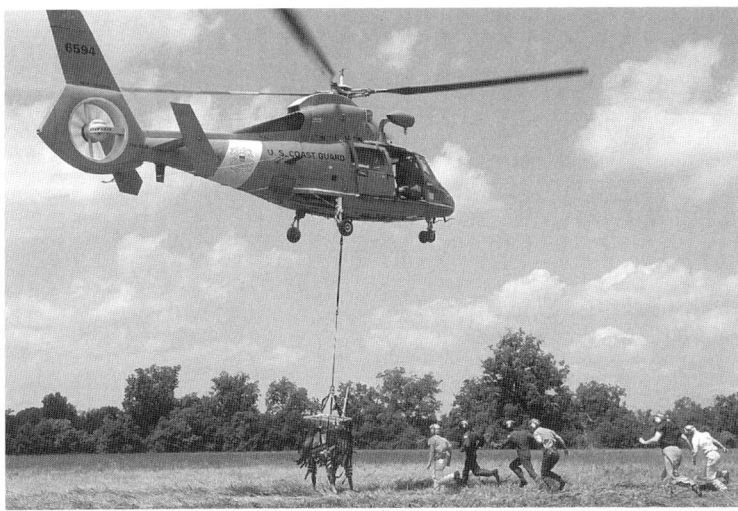

Fig. 5. Rescue of horse from flooded farm area in April 2001 during Tropical Storm Allison in Pineville, Louisiana. (*Courtesy of* Harry Cowgill, Baton Rouge, LA.)

sustained traumatic injury associated with fleeing the rescuers, and were difficult to restrain chemically and prepare for rescue. Eventually, all 16 horses were safely transported by boat using short-acting general anesthesia or an Anderson sling combined with Coast Guard helicopter rescue (Fig. 5) [6].

Equine emergency field response activities should be performed by an experienced team of individuals including veterinarians, first responders, and trained animal handlers to provide for safety of human beings and horses. With equine rescue, responders often get hurt and the horse may sustain more injury as a result of the rescue activities. A basic guideline is to use the simplest, safest, and most "low-tech" approach in an effort to minimize injury to the victims and rescuers [7]. Stressed and injured horses can be extremely unpredictable and can pose significant endangerment situations for people. Decisions regarding the appropriate type of response (whether it is rescue, field medical treatment, sheltering, or simply provision of feed and water) should be made with the safety of response personnel being a primary objective.

During the Hurricane Katrina aftermath response, the equine branch communications center received numerous calls from evacuees who wanted to know the status of their horses that had weathered the storm or had been evacuated to an area that had then received storm damage. Countless calls were received from people who simply wanted information on the status of something that they had seen on television, often hampering the calls from people with true needs. Equine branch communications center leaders were tasked with prioritizing numerous requests from equine owners (Fig. 6). Response plans were organized with intelligence received from the field about

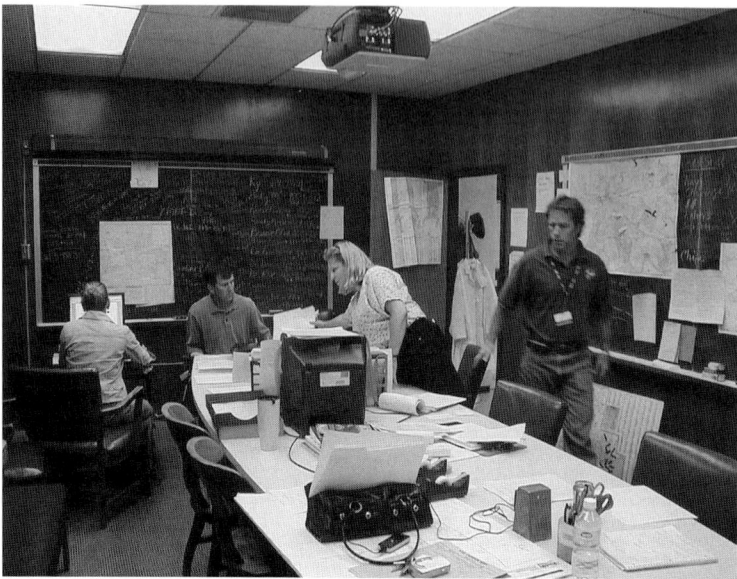

Fig. 6. Equine branch communications center at Louisiana State University, School of Veterinary Medicine, in September 2005 during the aftermath of Hurricanes Katrina and Rita.

known animals in need of rescue or urgent medical care and were then grouped into geographic location.

Triage and medical treatment

For horses stranded in a flood, stress is a major contributor to flood-related equine medical problems and can include colic, diarrhea, dehydration, neurologic disease, respiratory disease, laminitis, sole abscesses, skin abrasions, cellulitis, lacerations, fracture disease, and corneal injuries. The innate equine "fight or flight" response can often accentuate even minor medical problems into sometimes life-threatening situations. If possible, injured horses should be examined by a veterinarian in the field and medically stabilized before transport. Stabilization may include sedation to prevent further traumatic injury to the patient and handlers. Attempts to transport fractious patients can make the situation worse, especially if the horses are improperly restrained. Horses that are severely dehydrated or exhibiting signs of cardiovascular shock may benefit from large-volume bolus intravenous fluid therapy in the field before transport (isotonic polyionic fluids, 50 mL/kg administered intravenously initially, followed by 20–30 L per 450-kg adult horse). During heightened stressful situations, such as flood response and rescue, it is important to move the patient to an area for initial triage and assessment as soon as possible.

Equine flood victims should be decontaminated by bathing with detergent soap products and require thorough rinsing to remove toxins, debris, or microorganisms from the skin and to identify additional sites of injury. Recommended products for bathing include Dawn or Ivory dishwashing soap or human or animal shampoo products without additives. The underside of the hooves should be scrubbed clean and examined to determine if debris or hoof punctures can be identified.

Handling and restraint

Chemical restraint is often indicated to manage the rescue, medical evaluation, and treatment of flood-stranded horses safely. Chemical restraint can minimize further injury to the patient and prevent human injury as well as allowing rescue activities (including trailer extraction or helicopter sling rescue). Recommended chemical restraints include acetylpromazine (0.02–0.08 mg/kg administered intravenously), xylazine (0.5–0.75 mg/kg administered intravenously), detomidine (5–20 µg/kg administered intravenously), and butorphanol (0.01–0.02 mg/kg administered intravenously). Yohimbine (0.1–0.15 mg/kg administered intravenously) may be indicated for α_2-agonist reversal in the event of significant bradycardia and hypotension [8]. An adverse response to sedation and tranquilization can produce hypotension, decreased gastrointestinal motility, and exacerbation of cardiovascular shock. Several veterinarians experienced in equine rescue recommend detomidine sedation (5–20 µg/kg administered intravenously) followed by butorphanol (0.01–0.02 mg/kg administered intravenously) for airlift or trailer extraction [8]. Horses rescued by means of flat boats (pontoon boats) require general short-acting anesthesia using the "triple-drip" method (guaifenesin, ketamine, and detomidine) [9]. The horse or pony is typically premedicated with detomidine (10–20 µg/kg) and then induced with a ketamine (2 mg/kg) intravenous bolus; after induction, anesthesia is maintained using the triple drip (2 mL/kg/h). If a 15-drop/mL infusion set is used, the rate for administration of the triple-drip solution is 1 drop per second to maintain the horse under general anesthesia. Recovery usually occurs 35 to 40 minutes after discontinuing the infusion. It is critical to provide a safe area for recovery. This may be particularly challenging in a disaster flood environment.

Integument and musculoskeletal injury

Extremity, head, neck, and trunk lacerations and abrasions are commonly seen in equine flood victims. Limb lacerations are especially common and can involve fractures or tendon lacerations. A horse exhibiting moderate to severe lameness requires detailed examination to localize the lameness and prevent further exacerbation. Diagnostics should focus on blunt and penetrating traumatic injuries, which can result in bone fracture, soft tissue injury, nail penetration into the foot, or a combination of injuries. Access to splinting devices, such as lower limb protection using a Kimsey splint, is beneficial.

Flood-affected horses may develop dermatitis and cellulitis because of breeches in the skin's barrier capabilities from standing in contaminated water for long periods. Contaminants may include chemicals (eg, oil spill related), sewage, minerals (involving mining or rock quarries), elevated salinity (gulf, ocean, or brackish waters), or other substances. Flood waters with high saline levels are more likely to cause diseases associated with ingestion of water, such as colitis or neurologic disease. Mild to moderate cases of dermatitis and cellulitis can lead to more serious complications, such as septic tenosynovitis or septic arthritis, and if not treated aggressively, these infections can lead to severe lameness or loss of use, and some may even be life ending. Early recognition and diagnosis of cellulitis enable the rapid aggressive intervention necessary for a positive outcome. Delay in diagnosis and treatment increases complication and mortality rates and makes these conditions difficult to treat successfully. Horses with cellulitis have swelling and heat in affected areas. They show signs of pain and lameness and often have a low-grade fever (102°F–104°F). Horses with more severe infections become anorectic and show signs of serious discomfort. Their legs become extremely painful when touched, and they may show moderate to severe lameness of that limb. Systemic antimicrobial therapy is indicated in cases of cellulitis and should be based on broad-spectrum capabilities and tissue penetration. β-Lactam antimicrobials are indicated because of the risk of clostridial diseases and other anaerobic bacterial infections. Standard dosing of ceftiofur sodium (2.2 mg/kg administered intravenously or intramuscularly every 6 to 8 hours), procaine penicillin G (22,000 IU/kg administered intramuscularly every 12 hours), or penicillin G potassium (22,000 IU/kg administered intravenously every 6 hours) combined with an aminoglycoside and oral metronidazole (20–25 mg/kg administered per os or per rectum) offers excellent coverage of most bacterial organisms. Antimicrobial treatment for cellulitis should continue for 10 to 14 days and possibly longer if necessary.

Horses exposed to flood waters may be at higher risk of developing extremity dermatitis- and cellulitis-associated fungal or fungal-like diseases, such as equine Pythium or Basidiobolus. In horses, fungal skin infections can be invasive and rapidly progressive and can cause proliferative pyogranulomatous disease. Lesions can be ulcerative and oozing and may have a foul odor. The growing cutaneous mass might be especially pruritic, and affected animals often are stressed and agitated, which might lead to self-mutilation in an attempt to relieve the discomfort. Grossly, the lesions may be confused with exuberant granulation tissue. Fungal skin disease requires definitive diagnosis by means of a biopsy and fungal culture (Pythium Laboratory, Louisiana State

University, Baton Rouge, Lousiana) for determination of appropriate treatment [10]. If skin lacerations, dermatitis, and cellulitis fail to respond to standard care, including systemic antibacterial therapy, fungal infection needs to be ruled out by means of a skin biopsy for histopathology and fungal culture. Treatment includes a combination of surgery, antifungals, and immunotherapy.

Hoof problems

Horses that have been standing in mud or water for long periods may develop thrush, soft soles, and sloughing of the frog, which compromise the strength of the hooves' support structures and can make the horse more prone to sole bruising and other hoof problems. Once dry, their hooves may be more susceptible to separation of the laminae and to subsequent white line disease, laminitis, or foot abscessation. The horse's feet should be cleaned using a hoof pick and brush as soon as possible to remove sharp debris capable of puncturing the hoof wall or sole. Horses that have been standing in mud, water, or debris for extended periods may require medical farriery (podiatry) to treat thrush, hoof or sole defects, coronitis, or laminitis. Application of iodine-based hoof preparations toughens up soft soles and draws some of the moisture out of hooves that are too soft. Additionally, thrush-fighting products found in farm supply and tack stores can effectively treat minor cases of thrush if used appropriately.

Ophthalmic injuries

Ophthalmic injuries, especially traumatic corneal ulceration and uveitis, are common medical emergencies observed in equine flood victims as a result of flying storm debris and damaged stable and pasture environments. Animal handlers and first responders may not recognize ophthalmic injuries as they concentrate on more obvious injuries and participate in rescue activities. A thorough ophthalmic examination and early recognition and treatment are important for preventing more serious infections. Equine eyes should be irrigated with sterile eyewash solution, and the veterinarian should perform a close detailed ophthalmic examination, which requires sedation in most cases. The eye examination should include fluoroscein staining of both eyes to rule out the presence of traumatic corneal defects. Corneal abrasions and ulcers may quickly become bacterial or fungal infections if not treated preventatively and aggressively. Deep corneal invasion of fungi and concurrent bacterial infection can lead to corneal perforation and iris prolapse. Common clinical signs of fungal keratitis include ocular pain manifested by blepharospasm, epiphora or photophobia, fluorescein-positive corneal ulceration, or corneal neovascularization as well as and uveitis manifested by miosis and aqueous flare. Prevention of fungal keratitis should include topical treatment with antifungal agents, such as miconazole or silver sulfadiazine cream [11]. Broad-spectrum antibacterial agents include ophthalmic triple-antibiotic ointment, ciprofloxacin, and tobramycin. Atropine 1% ophthalmic solution or ointment should be applied topically as frequently as is necessary to maintain pupillary dilation in horses with storm-related traumatic corneal defects. Fungal infections may be difficult to treat; thus, early recognition and treatment are important to a successful outcome. Ocular pain may also be controlled by the systemic administration of nonsteroidal anti-inflammatory (NSAIDS) drugs, such as phenylbutazone (2.2 mg/kg every 12 to 24 hours) or flunixin meglumine (1.1 mg/kg every 12 to 24 hours) for 5 to 7 days, thereafter gradually reducing the dose to 50% or less. Corticosteroid therapy should not be included in treating traumatic corneal ulceration in the horse.

Gastrointestinal dysfunction

Horses that are stressed from being stranded, injured, or unattended during a flood situation or have ingested contaminated water, hay, or grain may develop colitis or another form of colic or systemic toxemia requiring moderate to aggressive medical care. Frequently, horses show signs of lethargy, inappetence, and colic, and some may develop mild to severe diarrhea. Physical examination may reveal an increased respiratory rate or heart rate attributable to abdominal discomfort as well as an increased rectal temperature attributable to toxin absorption. Signs of abdominal discomfort can range from mild (eg, recumbency, inappetence) to severe (eg, rolling, thrashing). There is often gross abdominal distention if the large colon is affected. Colitis may be confused with other large bowel disorders, including large colon torsion or volvulus, whereby surgical intervention may become necessary. Mucous membranes may be tacky with a delayed capillary refill time, and skin turgor may be reduced. Systemic absorption of endotoxin can result in peripheral arteriovenous shunting and classic "brick-red" mucous membranes. Hypovolemia and subsequent circulatory shock can cause purple mucous membranes and weak peripheral pulses.

Treatment regimens are supportive and aimed at plasma volume replacement (crystalloid fluid replacement), analgesia and anti-inflammatory therapy, antiendotoxin therapy, antimicrobial therapy if indicated, and nutritional support. Aggressive intravenous polyionic fluid therapy should be instituted immediately in horses showing signs of toxemia, colic, clinical dehydration, or colitis. Total fluid deficits should be calculated based on clinical assessment of dehydration (eg, for 8% or moderate dehydration, 0.08×450-kg body weight = 36 L), and replacement fluids should be administered rapidly (up to 6–10 L/h per 450-kg adult horse). Many horses with colic associated with dehydration and electrolyte imbalances voluntarily consume various types of electrolyte mixture. In addition to offering a fresh clean water source, offering mixtures of electrolytes in water may be beneficial in some cases. Mixtures to consider providing include water with baking soda (10 g/L), water with sodium chloride (NaCl) and potassium chloride (KCl) ("lite" salt) at a rate of 6 to 10 g/L, and water with a commercial electrolyte solution. Horses with nasogastric reflux should not be offered water until normal transit of fluid and ingesta is re-established. Horses with unrelenting signs of an abdominal crisis, including colitis, with a minimal clinical response should be referred to a veterinary facility capable of providing intensive care treatment or surgical intervention.

Horses with signs of toxemia (elevated heart rate, brick-red mucous membranes, and clinical dehydration) may have absorbed large amounts of endotoxin from a disrupted intestinal mucosal barrier, thus putting these horses at high risk for developing laminitis, thrombophlebitis, and disseminated intravascular coagulation. Specific treatment to combat endotoxemia is crucial for patient survival. The choice of treatment options is based on the severity of the disease, renal function, and hydration status as well as on economics. Antiendotoxin treatment target areas include (1) endotoxin neutralization before interaction with inflammatory cells; (2) prevention of the synthesis, release, or action of mediator activity; and (3) general supportive care (Table 1).

NSAIDs are the most frequently used group of drugs for treating abdominal pain in horses (flunixin meglumine, 1.1 mg/kg administered intravenously every 12 hours; phenylbutazone, 2.2 mg/kg administered per os or intravenously every 12 hours). The veterinarian must weigh the benefit of the analgesic effect of NSAIDs against the possibility of further damaging

Table 1
Antiendotoxin therapy

Product	Dosing information
Endoserum	1.5 mL/kg of body weight intravenously diluted at a 1:10 or 1:20 ratio in sterile isotonic saline or lactated Ringer's solution
Polymyxin B	1000–6000 IU/kg of body weight administered intravenously every 8–12 hours for up to 3 days. Because of the possibility of causing nephrotoxic side effects, polymyxin B should be used judiciously, and its use in azotemic patients is not recommended
Flunixin meglumine	0.25 mg/kg of body weight three or four times daily
Dimethylsulfoxide	0.1 g/kg of body weight administered intravenously (higher doses have been associated with exacerbating intestinal reperfusion injury in horses)
Allopurinol	5 mg/kg of body weight administered intravenously
Pentoxyphylline	8 mg/kg of body weight administered per os three times daily

the bowel by potentially blocking the protective effects of intestinal mucosal prostaglandins. Endogenous prostaglandins have been shown repeatedly to be important inhibitors of the development of intestinal inflammation, and blocking these with NSAIDs may slow the recovery and healing of inflamed cecal or colonic mucosa. Alternative choices for analgesia need to be considered. Butorphanol (an opioid analgesic, 0.06–0.1 mg/kg administered intramuscularly) combined with detomidine (an α–agonist, 0.01–0.02 mg/kg administered intramuscularly) every 6 to 8 hours is a useful combination that has minimal effects on gastrointestinal motility.

The use of broad-spectrum intravenous antibiotics in cases of colic and colitis is not always indicated. Mild and transient neutropenia or fever may not justify the use of broad-spectrum antimicrobials, but they should be considered when the patient has concurrent problems warranting treatment or profound or persistent neutropenia and may be at an increased risk for complications associated with sepsis, such as peritonitis, pneumonia, cellulitis, thrombophlebitis, or coagulation dysfunction. Potassium penicillin (22,000 IU/kg administered every 6 hours) in combination with gentamicin (4.4–6.6 mg/kg administered every 24 hours) is a commonly used therapy in these cases. Oral broad-spectrum antimicrobial medications are not recommended because they may further disrupt the intestinal microbial population. Oral metronidazole (15–25 mg/kg administered every 8 hours) may be indicated in cases in which *Clostridium* spp are suspected as playing a role in the pathogenesis of the disease. In addition, metronidazole may have local anti-inflammatory effects and may be effective in treating acute equine colitis of unknown cause. Treatment with metronidazole has been associated with causing anorexia in some horses [12]. Effective antisecretory medications targeting the equine large colon have not been identified. It is unlikely that bismuth subsalicylate or similar protectant agents are effective for treating large-bowel diarrhea in the adult horse because of the large volume of large intestinal contents. Horses with diarrhea may benefit from treatment with oral adsorbents, such as activated charcoal or smectite powder. Nasogastric intubation with mineral oil may promote resolution of intestinal impaction colic and may inhibit absorption of toxins through the damaged intestinal mucosal barrier. Nutritional needs of horses with resolving colic and colitis are an important consideration. Flood-affected and injured horses often have a ravenous appetite and should be allowed to eat judicious amounts of good-quality hay and fresh green grass (if available). Fresh water should be provided in small amounts initially and then ad libitum. Re-establishment of normal feeding and watering should occur over 48 to 72 hours.

Neurologic disease

Equine flood victims are at increased risk of developing head and neck injuries and are more susceptible to infectious diseases, such as viral encephalitides or clostridial infections (tetanus and botulism). During patient triage, initial physical examination findings suggestive of central neurologic disease require immediate action to prevent further progression of neurologic abnormalities. Vaccination with tetanus toxoid is indicated if the vaccination status of the patient is unknown. Vaccinating against encephalitides or viral and bacterial respiratory diseases may be contraindicated, because the immune response in an extremely stressed horse is minimal and may actually contribute to a raised stress level in equine flood victims [13]. In hindsight, there was a general consensus from Hurricane Katrina and Rita equine response veterinarians that tetanus vaccine was indicated for animals rescued because of their increased risk for this potentially life-threatening disease but that vaccinating extremely stressed horses with respiratory and encephalitis vaccines was not effective and may have contributed to the adverse reactions observed in a few of the horses.

If ingested water contains elevated saline levels, such as waters contaminated with coastal storm surge, veterinarians treating potentially salt-intoxicated horses must be judicious with administration of intravenous or oral fluids to prevent exacerbation of potential salt toxicity. Ingestion of water containing total dissolved salt at a rate more than 7000 mg/L has the potential to cause acute salt poisoning. Salt poisoning may occur secondary to water deprivation, which may happen when horses are left unattended for several consecutive days. This was the case for several dozen horses during the aftermath of Hurricane Katrina. With the looting and civil unrest that ensued 3 to 5 days after the storm's landfall and the declaration of martial law in the Greater New Orleans area, rescue teams were denied access to these animals for 3 to 5 additional days and many horses were found to have been locked in their stalls in ankle to knee-deep mud without access to potable water for up to 7 days. Detailed specific management of salt poisoning in horses is covered elsewhere. The basic principles include prevention by replenishing plasma volume hydration more slowly than in standard cases of hypovolemia as well as close monitoring of serum sodium or osmolality and clinical neurologic signs. Treatment with systemic anti-inflammatory medications may help to minimize signs of cerebral edema.

Respiratory disease

Aspiration of water in horses exposed to flood waters may cause acute pulmonary edema and pneumonia, which is usually life threatening. Even small amounts of aspiration may lead to inflammation and consolidation of the lungs. Secondary bacterial invasion is likely, and if the horse survives acute insults, this could later develop into severe septic pneumonia or pleuropneumonia. Horses that have been found to be stranded or "stuck" in ponds, deep mud, or flood waters and struggle and flail for long periods can develop upper respiratory tract inflammation (eg, chondritis, pharyngitis, laryngitis). Emergency tracheotomy may be necessary in horses that have developed URT obstruction secondary to long periods of struggling. Aspiration pneumonia may occur secondary to laryngeal dysfunction. Treatment includes aggressive anti-inflammatory therapy, systemic broad-spectrum antibiotics, and, if the horse is not dehydrated, furosemide to address pulmonary edema.

Horses that are evacuated or rescued after a flood event may be commingled and become infected with respiratory infections, such as equine influenza, rhinopneumonitis, or *Streptococcus equi*. Herd health programs aimed at providing herd immunity optimization before storm seasons can help to minimize herd outbreaks in the event of such a situation.

Summary

Of the nearly 500 horses evacuated, rescued, and sheltered in Louisiana after Hurricanes Katrina and Rita, most were only mildly affected and seemed to need only the "basics" of solid dry footing, food, and clean drinking water. There is no way to prepare for every situation that arises in a disaster. By working closely with other producers and agricultural leaders, however, horse owners can lessen the impact of a disaster on their operation. Preparation and detailed planning are the most important aspects of flood-related injury prevention. Encouraging animal owners and caretakers to have an evacuation plan and dispersing knowledge about local and regional disaster authorities are critical for a successful disaster response. Educational programs on future disaster response empower communities to care for their people and animals responsibly.

References

[1] Flood hazards: a national threat (fact sheet). Available at: http://pubs.usgs.gov/fs/2006/3026/. Accessed November 20, 2006.
[2] Available at: http://animalid.aphis.usda.gov/nais/downloads/print/EquineNAIS_Informational_Booklet6-06.pdf. Accessed November 20, 2006.
[3] Available at: http://nc.sartusa.org/. Accessed November 20, 2006.
[4] Available at: http://www.cosart.org/. Accessed November 20, 2006.
[5] Available at: http://www.LSART.org. Accessed November 20, 2006.
[6] Pettifer G, Smith J, McConnico RS, et al. Airlifting horses by helicopter: sedation requirements. 26th Annual Meeting of the American College of Veterinary Anesthesiologists held in New Orleans, October 11–12, 2001. Veterinary Anaesthesiology Analg 2002;29:108.
[7] Gimenez T, Gimenez RM, Baker JL, et al. How to effectively perform emergency rescue of equines. Proceedings of the American Association of Equine Practitioners 2002;48:276–81.
[8] Madigan JE. Rescue of the individual horse. Proceedings of the American Association of Equine Practitioners, 1993;38:141–4.
[9] van Dijk P. Intravenous anaesthesia in horses by guaiphenesin-ketamine-detomidine infusion: some effects. Vet Q 1994;16(Suppl 2):S122–4.
[10] Grooters AM, Whittington A, Lopez MK, et al. Evaluation of microbial culture techniques for the isolation of Pythium insidiosum from equine tissues. J Vet Diagn Invest 2002;14(4):288–94.

[11] Cutler TJ. Corneal epithelial disease. Vet Clin North Am Equine Pract 2004;20(2):319–43.
[12] Sweeney RW, CR, Weiher J. Clinical use of metronidazole in horses: 200 cases (1984–1989). J Am Vet Med Assoc 1991;198(6):1045–48.
[13] Folsom RW, Littlefield-Chabaud MA, French DD, et al. Exercise alters the immune response to equine influenza virus and increases susceptibility to infection. Equine Vet J 2001;33(7):664–9.

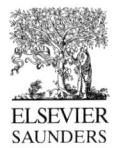

Fire and Smoke Inhalation Injury in Horses

Peggy S. Marsh, DVM

Department of Large Animal Clinical Sciences, College of Veterinary Medicine, Texas A&M University, 4475 TAMU, College Station, TX 77843-4475, USA

Exposure to fire and smoke can cause devastating traumatic injury. In general, providing medical management of this type of injury is not common for the equine veterinarian. Much of the information about such types of injury has been generated by research related to human injury. Although the incidence of burn injuries in people is on the decline in the United State, there are still 1 to 2 million people treated for burns annually [1–3]. Most of the injuries are minor; however, 20,000 to 50,000 people require hospital care. The most severely affected patients are treated in specialized burn units, wherein the fatality rate is approximately 4% [1,3]. Although trauma from fires, with or without concurrent smoke inhalation injury, in horses is comparatively quite low (with no information reported on the incidence), when it does occur, the results are typically tragic. Sporadic reports of barn fires most commonly note high mortality, with few, if any, horses removed alive from burning buildings. Although large wildfires make national news, there is limited information on the number of horses affected and the types of injuries that occur.

The injuries that horses incur after being exposed to fire or smoke can range from mild to severe, with multiple body systems involved. Thermal injury to the surface produces one of the most prominent types of lesions affecting these victims, and in human medicine, estimation of the extent and depth of burn injury is an important aspect in the initial management [3]. Classification systems based on the depth of injury are routinely used in human medicine and have been extrapolated to horses [4,5].

Respiratory tract lesions are also common in these types of patients and can require emergency therapy. In addition to these more familiar types of lesions, fire and smoke trauma can produce numerous physiologic responses,

E-mail address: pmarsh@cvm.tamu.edu

and depending on the severity, the systemic response can be life threatening. Significant systemic involvement is termed *burn shock*, and one of the most striking features is the development of severe edema. The wide variety of possible body systems that can be involved can make these cases challenging to manage medically.

The role of an equine emergency veterinarian in these situations can be varied, ranging from being part of the first-response team, to providing care to critically ill individuals, to helping clients be as prepared as possible for such types of disasters. The goal of this article is to provide a basic review on the pathophysiology of fire and smoke injury as well as to discuss diagnostic and therapeutic goals to aid the practitioner when he or she is faced with such a potentially overwhelming and emotionally charged situation.

First response and disaster preparedness

The two most common ways for horses to receive fire and smoke injury are by being trapped within a burning barn or being in the path of a wildfire. Expected types of injuries vary in each of these situations. In general, barn fires occur with no warning; depending on the material of the barn, the fire can consume the building rapidly, with only several minutes to move animals out. If one is part of the first-response team, it is imperative to follow all instructions of fire control personnel. Entering a burning building is highly dangerous, and it is difficult to predict how an animal is going to react in such situations. Disaster planning is becoming more widespread, and a search of the Internet yields several horse protection groups conducting training sessions specific to removing horses from a burning barn. Practices seen in movies, such as covering the horse's eyes, may not work and may cause more panic in some situations.

As part of the first-response team, a veterinarian may be most productive by focusing attention on the animals removed from the fire. At first, these animals may not outwardly show the extent of their injuries, dermally or systemically. Initially, the goal should be to stop the burning processes [6]. Remove any blankets or wraps that can continue to hold heat next to the animal. Cooling of the patient to limit thermal injury could be considered within the first few minutes with the use of lukewarm water [6]. Causing vasoconstriction of poorly perfused hypoxic tissue by using ice or extremely cold water is contraindicated, however [7]. Primary treatment should be limited to that needed to stabilize the patient and, most commonly, would include sedation to minimize excitement and anti-inflammatory drugs. Also, if feasible, securing intravenous access might be considered during this initial evaluation. Substantial edema can occur within hours, making venous access difficult. After a complete physical examination, movement of an affected horse to a location where further diagnostic evaluation and intensive treatment can occur is recommended. Because exposure to hypoxic conditions has most likely occurred, availability of oxygen therapy is ideal.

There is little to no information specific to the types of injuries that horses incur when they are in the path of a wildfire. In general, smoke inhalation injury would be expected to be less common, and in addition to thermal injury to the body surface, cuts and contusions might be seen in animals left to fend for themselves. Moving across hot surfaces may also cause thermal damage to the solar surface of hooves. Although wildfires can move rapidly under the right conditions, there is often time for evacuation. Helping clients who live in high-risk areas to create a rational plan, including helping them to develop a transport plan with information on safe holding locations as well as on providing permanent identification, would be useful. Veterinarians who practice in high-risk areas often play a vital role in community disaster planning activities.

Pathophysiology of fire injury

The type and extent of injury depend on factors related to the fire as well as on the duration of exposure and location of the victim relative to the point of origin of the fire. Thermal injury causes a local response that includes microvascular insult and direct tissue coagulation, leading to local inflammation, edema, and, finally, necrosis. Extensive local injuries drive a systemic response. The initial systemic response is attributable, in part, to loss of the skin barrier as well as to release of multiple mediators that can initiate the inflammatory and coagulation cascades [2]. The effects of hypoxia and subsequent reperfusion injury on various organs and tissue beds can complicate recovery from severe thermal trauma [8].

Initially, there is a decrease in cardiac output; however, in focally damaged areas, there is an increase in capillary pressures. These characteristics, which are typical in early shock, represent the initial phase of burn shock. Directly after these changes, there is formation of generalized edema. The pathophysiology of burn edema is complex and involves endothelial damage, protein shifts, and alteration of the interstitial architecture. All these factors lead to a net accumulation of fluid in the interstitial spaces [9]. In addition to the changes incited by direct thermal injury, release of various mediators plays an important role in edema formation. Some of the most prominent mediators include neutrophils, which are a known source of oxidants, as well as prostaglandins, bradykinins, and histamines. Oxidants are produced as a result of focal tissue hypoxia, followed by reperfusion. The results of reperfusion injury cause endothelial cell damage as well as denaturation and fragmentation of interstitial matrix components [9]. Prostacyclin and thromboxane are reported to be detected in burn edema [9]. Although they have opposite effects (prostacyclin is a vasodilator, and thromboxane has vasoconstrictive activities), when expressed in locally damaged tissues, both contribute to cardiovascular instability and edema formation. Bradykinins and histamines are known to increase vascular permeability. Edema develops not only in tissue directly affected by thermal injury but is seen at distant sites when the burn size exceeds approximately 20% of the body surface [2].

In the long run, high cardiac output, insulin resistance, and increased oxygen consumption with protein and fat wasting, all of which may create a hypermetabolic state, characterize major thermal injury [2,10,11]. Endogenous catecholamines have been implicated as the initiating mediators of this hypermetabolic response [12]. Loss of skin as a barrier, release of inflammatory mediators, and hypermetabolism play a role in the development of immunosuppression. Systemic changes may lead to gastrointestinal tract dysfunction, and disruption of this system can lead to bacterial translocation, increasing the risk of significant infections [13]. Other features noted with burn injury in the horse include anemia secondary to acute hemolysis, renal failure, laminitis, and myositis [14].

Pathophysiology of inhalation injury

The combination of thermal injury with smoke inhalation is known to result in increased morbidity and mortality in human patients [9,15,16]. In closed burning buildings, victims close to the point of origin are more likely to be overcome by direct thermal injury, whereas others at some distance may incur injuries as a result of smoke inhalation [17]. There are infrequent reports of horse with primary smoke inhalation injury [18,19]. The pathophysiology of smoke inhalation injury is complex and multifactorial. Insult to the respiratory system by smoke inhalation depends on the fuels that burned, completeness of combustion, and generated heat intensity.

There are three primary mechanisms of injury: direct thermal effects, toxic gas effects, and hypoxia. Similar to thermal injury of the skin, edema formation is a key component of the initial respiratory injury. Direct thermal injury to the respiratory tract can be limited to the upper respiratory tract by laryngeal reflexes and efficient heat exchange within the nasal passages. Toxic chemicals in the smoke can cause damage, directly and indirectly, through inflammatory mediators. Carbon monoxide intoxication is commonly associated with human injuries from smoke and is a product of incomplete combustion [20]. Newer synthetic building materials contain other potential toxins, and forensic fire investigations have revealed that hydrogen cyanide is likely to be present in appreciable amounts in the blood of fire victims [17]. Finally, with combustion, there is consumption of oxygen, and the resulting low Pao_2 can lead to pulmonary vasoconstriction as well as generalized hypoxia.

Three phases of pulmonary dysfunction have been described in the horse [4,18]. The first stage is acute pulmonary insufficiency caused by several mechanisms. Carbon monoxide may be present in a sufficiently high concentration to cause toxicity within a short time after exposure. Carbon monoxide combines with hemoglobin to form carboxyhemoglobin, which reduces the circulating oxygen-carrying capacity. Hemoglobin has a 200 to 250 times greater affinity for carbon monoxide as compared with its affinity for oxygen [20]. High levels of circulating carboxyhemoglobin result in a shift of the oxyhemoglobin dissociation curve to the left, thereby decreasing oxygen release at the tissue level and leading to tissue hypoxia. Carbon monoxide can also combine with myoglobin, leading to impaired diffusion of oxygen to muscles [17]. Other processes occurring during this acute phase include progressive edema and necrosis in the upper respiratory tract leading to airway obstruction, bronchoconstriction in the lower respiratory tract from the irritating effects of noxious products, and altered pulmonary blood flow [15,16].

These insults produce the second stage, which includes the formation of pulmonary edema, lower airway obstruction, and pulmonary parenchymal lesions. Within 24 to 72 hours after exposure, driven by pulmonary macrophages, neutrophils are called into the area of insult. They release cytokines, proteolytic enzymes, and oxygen-derived free radicals. Expression of the inflammatory cascade in excess of balance causes microvascular damage, leading to increased extravascular lung water. Local insult also results in the release of tissue factor initiating the coagulation cascade to produce fibrin. Debris from the inflammatory cascade, along with fibrin and material directly deposited from smoke inhalation, creates pseudomembranous casts, which may obstruct the small airways. Widespread plugging of the airways may significantly increase airway pressure, causing barotrauma and alveolar damage [15]. Bronchopneumonia is the last stage and occurs as a result of the impaired host immune system, locally and systemically. This phase, if it occurs, may take up to 1 to 2 weeks after the initial injury to become clinically apparent.

Clinical signs

Horses exposed to fire with smoke have a variety of clinical signs depending on the duration and type of exposure and the length of time from the insult. Initially, the extent of damage to the skin may be difficult to ascertain. Horses rescued from burning barns most commonly incur thermal injury of the head and dorsum. At first, the damage may not be clinically visible or may show as singed areas with a leather-type appearance (Fig. 1). Over the first 24 to 48 hours, surfaces affected by direct thermal injury often become edematous. The degree of local edema depends, in part, on the elasticity of the skin and surrounding tissues. Typically, this is limited along the dorsum of the horse, and the extent of injury may not be fully realized for days to weeks (Figs. 2 and 3). Blepharospasm and epiphora are commonly present and often indicate corneal damage (Fig. 4).

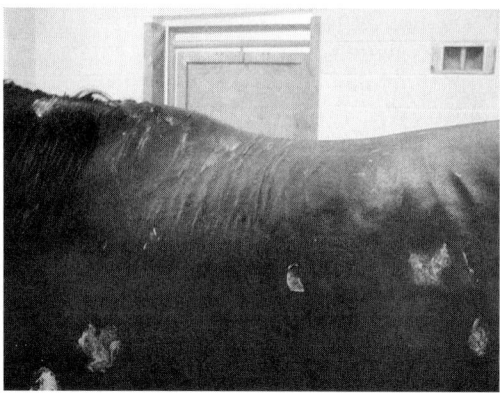

Fig. 1. Initial thermal injury along the back of a horse rescued from a barn fire. Note the smaller focal singed areas as well as the generalized leather-like appearance with hair loss across the back.

Depending on the depth of surface injury, sensation may be altered to these areas. In general, more superficial burn injuries cause more pain than deeper injuries, in which permanent damage to cutaneous sensation can occur. Altered sensation or pruritus associated with healing lesions can cause some horse to rub and self-traumatize damaged areas. A complication of successful long-term outcome in human injury includes the formation of restrictive scars. There are limited data on long-term outcomes in horses; however, extensive scar formation along the dorsum of an equine patient would certainly affect future use.

Acutely, within the first 6 hours, clinical signs of shock may be noted and include tachycardia, tachypnea, and altered mucous membrane color. It is during this period that the effect, if any, of carbon monoxide toxicosis may become clinically apparent. The patient may show signs of severe hypoxemia, which is evident by depression, disorientation, irritability, ataxia, or even a moribund to comatose status. As edema and necrosis progress in the upper respiratory tract, dyspnea and stridor may develop. Auscultation of the thorax may reveal decreased air movement, crackles, or wheezes, but these changes may not become apparent for 12 to 24 hours. If edema of the airways is sufficiently severe, air flow may be severely restricted. Edema fluid may be visible at the nostrils and, later, may be replaced by inflammatory exudate. During this same period, concurrent generalized edema may be forming.

Severely affected patients that are successfully resuscitated may start to show clinical improvement with stabilization of vital signs; however, secondary hypoxia in multiple tissue beds and generalized edema may lead to dysfunction of distant organs, such as the kidneys and muscles. It may take several days for organ dysfunction to become clinically apparent. Signs of infection may be difficult to differentiate from clinical signs of other

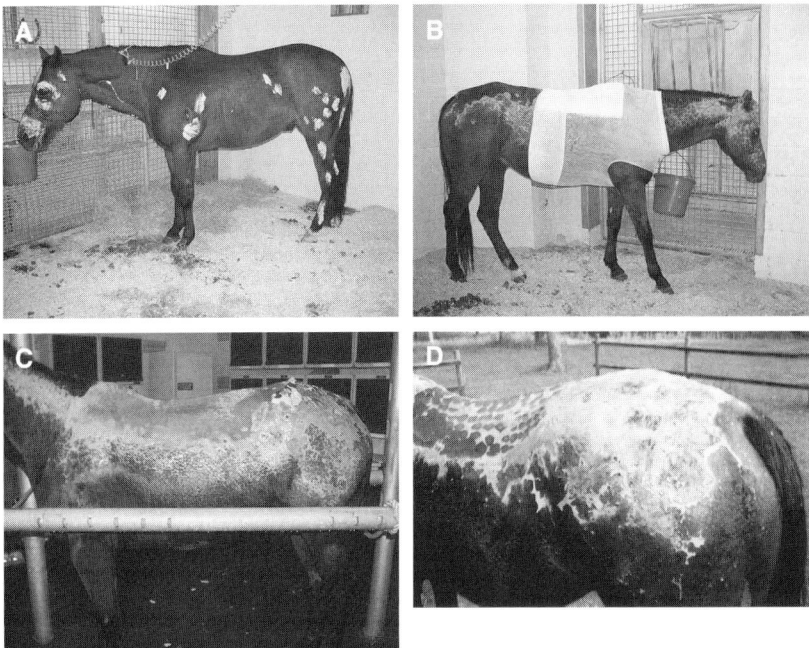

Fig. 2. This series of photographs documents the progression of thermal injury. This horse was rescued from a barn fire. Initially, it is difficult to ascertain the extent of the lesions. (*A*) At 24 hours after the trauma, edema of the muzzle and singed areas are noted as the most striking features. (*B, C*) Same patient at 6 and 20 weeks after injury. (*D*) Approximately 1 year after injury, the patient continues to require wound care. Note the black circles over the dorsal thorax, which are coalescing areas of healing skin grafts. Further resolution for this patient was obtained by the use of multiple punch skin grafts, with the exception of an area over the left gluteal muscles. Hot and humid conditions predisposed this individual to self-trauma of this region.

problems, and severely burned patients are at an increased risk of significant infection for a prolonged period. It is imperative to be vigilant for worsening of clinical signs after initial improvement as well as to monitor the horse for fever as an indication of possible infection.

Long term, the effects of a hypermetabolic response may become clinically evident as loss of body mass. Human patients with 40% body surface burn area can lose a quarter of their weight, even in the face of vigorous enteral alimentation [10]. In horses, this may be exhibited as those individuals that seem to waste away rapidly despite maintaining a good appetite. Healing of burn wound depends on depth and surface area affected. Even with aggressive surgical and medical management, large deep wounds can take prolonged time to heal and there is often scarring. Because many of the wounds involve the horse's back, it is important to remember that scarring can prevent future use of the equine patient for riding.

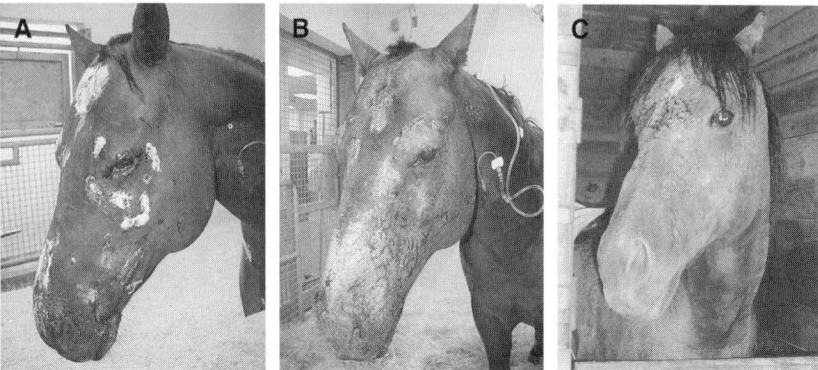

Fig. 3. Burn injury of the head is a common location for lesions. This series reveals clinical changes in lesions of the head in the same patient as in Fig. 2. There is a significant increase in the amount of edema present from the time of the photograph in *A*, which was taken within 6 hours of injury, to that in *B*, which was obtained 48 hours after the trauma. (*C*) Resolution of the lesions around the head occurred approximately 1 year later.

Diagnosis

Diagnosis is typically based on history and physical examination. A normal initial examination does not rule out exposure, because the onset of clinical signs may be delayed for several days. In human burn trauma, determining the extent of the surface area affected and the depth of the injury is an important diagnostic tool. Such information is useful to help determine the type of care required and for prognostic purposes. There are several protocols used to estimate the surface area, such as the "Rules of Nines" or the Lund and Browder charts [3]. There are also diagnostic techniques for determining the depth of injury, including biopsy and laser Doppler perfusion imaging. Even though a variety of theoretic methods

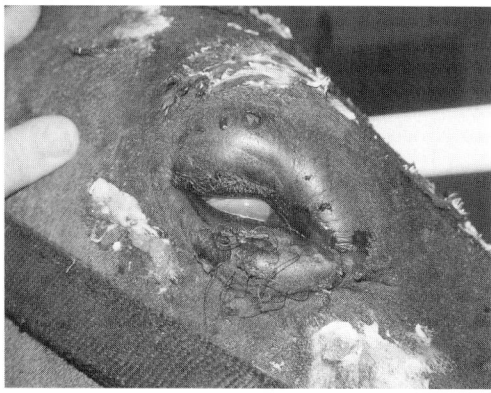

Fig. 4. Evidence of corneal trauma noted immediately in a horse rescued from a barn fire.

exist, this area is still an inexact science with human trauma. Again, there is limited information specific for the horse.

Diagnostic tools useful to judge the severity of cardiovascular compromise include blood pressure monitoring, measuring central venous pressure, serial lactate measurements, and monitoring urine production. Protein loss is thought to be a key component in edema formation; therefore, monitoring albumin levels as well as colloid oncotic pressure would be useful. Serial hematologic and serum chemistry analyses may be helpful to evaluate for dysfunction of various organ systems, such as renal failure or hemolytic anemia.

Various diagnostic tests are useful in determining the extent of respiratory injury. These include endoscopy of the upper respiratory tract and tracheobronchial tree, thoracic radiographs, blood gas analysis, hematology, and cytologic evaluation of tracheal aspirates. Any or all of these tests can be performed on a serial basis as prognostic aids. Within a short time after exposure, carboxyhemoglobin concentration in venous blood can be measured directly with a spectrophotometer. Serum levels fall rapidly; thus, evaluation for carboxyhemoglobin should occur as close as possible to the time of exposure. A level greater than 10% is consistent with carbon monoxide toxicity in the horse [4]. Carboxyhemoglobin and oxyhemoglobin reflect at the same wavelength; thus, pulse oximetry cannot be used to diagnosis carbon monoxide toxicity [21].

Treatment goals and prognosis

Treatment depends on the stage of injury. The initial therapeutic goals, as described previously, are to stop the burn process and gain intravenous access. Therapy should then be directed at improving or maintaining cardiovascular homeostasis. Intravenous fluid administration is the cornerstone of initial resuscitation of burn shock victims. Volumes required vary and should be tailored to the individual's needs based on clinical response. Monitoring urine output is a reasonable indicator of organ perfusion. A balanced polyionic electrolyte fluid is most commonly used. The use of a colloid during the initial phase of shock is controversial in human burn trauma. Some burn trauma centers tend to use colloid administration 12 to 24 hours after injury when the endothelial integrity may be returning to normal. Colloids like hydroxyethyl starch and fresh-frozen plasma have been described in treating equine patients [5]. The use of hypertonic saline to mobilize water from cells that may be overaccumulating fluid holds intuitive appeal; however, careful monitoring of sodium levels is required, and a recent study using hypertonic saline in burn shock revealed an increased incidence of renal failure and death [22].

Other therapeutic goals during the acute phase of burn shock include attenuation of inflammatory mediators and the use of free radical scavengers to treat reperfusion injury. Drugs like flunixin meglumine and pentoxifylline have been proposed for the inhibition of prostaglandins and tumor necrosis factor, respectively. Dimethyl sulfoxide (DMSO) and acetylcysteine are examples of medications that have been used to treat oxidative stress. Use of corticosteroids for the treatment of burn shock is not recommended for human injury and is controversial in equine patients because of the potential for immunosuppression and laminitis [4].

Attention to the respiratory system is also important in the acute phase. Oxygen support is of benefit. It is a treatment for carbon dioxide toxicity and helps to reduce hypoxemia [19]. Humidified oxygen can be supplied by nasal insufflation or by means of a transtracheal catheter. Upper respiratory tract obstruction may require a tracheostomy. Attention should be paid to keeping the airways clear, and nebulization may be useful, especially when pseudomembranous casts are suspected. Bronchodilators may be useful in counteracting reflex bronchoconstriction. Decreasing inflammation and pulmonary edema may require the use of diuretics and nonsteroidal anti-inflammatory drugs.

Burn wound management is complex, and the details are beyond the scope of this article. A recent report discusses the details of wound care management [5]. Topical antimicrobial therapy is used to help protect damaged areas from infection during the healing phase. Silver sulfadiazine is the most widely used topical treatment in burn patients, and this medication has been used in horses. A possible effect of this topical treatment, especially if used over large areas, is the development of leukopenia. When large areas of skin are damaged, there is loss of effective thermoregulation, and environmental temperatures should be controlled if possible. To help prevent infection, strict hygiene, meticulous nursing care, and optimal nutritional support should be provided [1,5]. Prophylactic systemic antimicrobial use is not recommended in human patients. Documented infection should be treated with appropriate antimicrobial agents based on the results of culture and sensitivity patterns [5].

Although it can be difficult to differentiate signs of pain from the clinical signs of shock, developing a comprehensive pain management plan is recommended. In addition to the use of nonsteroidal anti-inflammatory drugs, other options include opioid medications, such as morphine and butorphanol [23]. Lidocaine and ketamine have also been described for use in pain management in the horse [24,25]. All these medications can be administered as continuous rate infusions as needed. Providing a high-caloric and well-balanced diet is vital, and to help maintain healthy gastrointestinal function, the enteral route is preferred. Human patients with a hypermetabolic response require 1.4 to 2 times the resting energy requirements [10]. In the equine patient, supplementing high-quality hay and grain with energy-rich fat, such as vegetable oil, can meet these needs.

Novel therapies may include inhalation treatment with medications to inhibit inflammatory mediators, coagulation factors, or oxidative stress. This is useful in patients with significant respiratory dysfunction associated with plugging of airways. Treatments used have included inhalation of heparin, pentoxifylline, or acetylcysteine [26–28]. Another area of active research is the development of strategies to reduce catabolic effects of the hypermetabolic response. The use of medications, such as long-term propanolol, to block the β-adrenergic effects stimulated by high catecholamine levels has been helpful [29,30].

In the care of severely affected equine patients, it can be medically challenging to manage the multiple issues that can occur with fire- and smoke-associated trauma. Also, treatment of burn wounds can be prolonged and may require a lifetime of care with some individuals. During the initial emotional trauma in clients faced with such events, it is important to discuss the possible duration and cost of extended therapy as well as the chances of scar formation. There is no information on the long-term outcome of treatment of horses, especially in regard to the amount of surface area or depth of thermal injury. Although it may be possible to resuscitate the severely affected patient, it should be noted that euthanasia may be a reasonable option for patients with significant burn injury.

Summary

Fire and smoke can produce horrific traumatic injuries, and when such events involve horses, there is often high mortality. In addition to personal loss, there is often an emotional public response. Equine practitioners may be called on to perform several different types of services, ranging from being at the scene, to providing medical management, to helping with disaster plan development. Although injury may be mild, severe trauma can lead to complex critical cases with multiple organ system involvement that are a challenge to manage. Published information on these types of injuries specific to horses is limited. The extent of direct thermal injury may not be clinically evident initially. Severely affected equine patients may be successfully resuscitated but still face a poor prognosis because of the extent of dermal injuries.

References

[1] Monafo W. Initial management of burns. N Engl J Med 1996;335(21):1581–6.
[2] Sheridan R. Burns. Crit Care Med 2002;30(11):S500–14.
[3] Atiyeh BS, Gunn SW, Hayek SN. State of the art in burn treatment. World J Surg 2005;29(2): 131–48.
[4] Geor RJ, Ames TR. Smoke inhalation injury in horses. Compendium on Continuing Education for the Practicing Veterinarian 1991;13:1162–8.
[5] Hanson RR. Management of burn injuries in the horse. Vet Clin North Am Equine Pract 2005;21(1):105–23.
[6] Allison K, Porter K. Consensus on the pre-hospital approach to burns patient management. Injury, International Journal of the Care of the Injured 2004;35:734–8.

[7] Benson A, Dickson WA, Boyce DE. ABC of wound healing—burns. BMJ 2006;332:649–52.
[8] Sakurai H, Traber LD, Traber DL. Altered systemic organ blood flow after combined injury with burn and smoke inhalation. Shock 1998;9(5):369–74.
[9] Demling RH. The burn edema process: current concepts. J Burn Care Rehabil 2005;26(3): 207–27.
[10] Herndon DN, Tompkins RG. Support of the metabolic response to burn injury. Lancet 2004;363:1895–902.
[11] Pereira CT, Herndon DN. The pharmacologic modulation of the hypermetabolic response to burns. Adv Surg 2005;39:245–61.
[12] Wilmore DW, Long JN, Mason AD, et al. Catecholamines: mediator of the hypermetabolic response to thermal injury. Ann Surg 1974;180:653–69.
[13] Magnotti LJ, Deitch EA. Burns, bacterial translocation, gut barrier function, and failure. J Burn Care Rehabil 2005;26(5):383–91.
[14] Norman TE, Chaffin MK, Johnson MC, et al. Intravascular hemolysis associated with severe cutaneous burn injuries in five horses. J Am Vet Med Assoc 2005;226(12):2039–43.
[15] Murakami K, Tabor DL. Pathophysiological basis of smoke inhalation injury. News Physiol Sci 2003;18:125–9.
[16] Enkhbaatar P, Traber DL. Pathophysiology of acute lung injury in combined burn and smoke inhalation injury. Clin Sci 2004;107:137–43.
[17] Alarie Y. Toxicity of fire smoke. Crit Rev Toxicol 2002;32(4):259–89.
[18] Kirkland KD, Goetz TE, Foreman JH, et al. Smoke inhalation injury in a pony. Journal of Veterinary Emergency and Critical Care 1992;3:83–9.
[19] Kemper T, Spier S, Barratt-Boyes SM, et al. Treatment of smoke inhalation in five horses. J Am Vet Med Assoc 1993;202(7):91–4.
[20] Ernst A, Zibrak JD. Carbon monoxide poisoning. N Engl J Med 2003;339(22):1603–8.
[21] Marino PL. Oximetry and capnography. In: Marino PL, editor. The ICU book. Baltimore (MD): Williams and Wilkins; 1998. p. 355–70.
[22] Huang PP, Stucky FS, Dimick AR, et al. Hypertonic sodium resuscitation is associated with renal failure and death. Ann Surg 1995;221:543–54.
[23] Sellon DC, Monroe VL, Roberts MC, et al. Pharmacokinetics and adverse effects of butorphanol administered by single intravenous injection or continuous intravenous infusion in horses. Am J Vet Res 2001;62(2):183–9.
[24] Fielding CL, Brumbaugh GW, Matthews NS, et al. Pharmacokinetics and clinical effects of a subanesthetic continuous rate infusion of ketamine in awake horses. Am J Vet Res 2006; 67(9):1484–90.
[25] Malone E, Graham L. Management of gastrointestinal pain. Vet Clin North Am Equine Pract 2002;18(1):133–58.
[26] Tasaki O, Mozingo DW, Dubick MA, et al. Effects of heparin and lisofylline on pulmonary function after smoke inhalation injury in an ovine model. Crit Care Med 2002;30:637–43.
[27] Ogura H, Cioffi WG, Okerberg CV, et al. The effects of pentoxifylline on pulmonary function following smoke inhalation. J Surg Res 1994;56:242–50.
[28] Desai MH, Mlcak R, Richardson J, et al. Reduction in mortality in pediatric patients with inhalation injury with aerosolized heparin/acetylcysteine therapy. J Burn Care Rehabil 1998; 19:210–2.
[29] Herndon DN, Barrow RE, Rutan TC, et al. Effect of propranolol administration on hemodynamic and metabolic responses of burned pediatric patients. Ann Surg 1988;208:484–92.
[30] Baron PW, Barrow RE, Pierre EJ, et al. Prolonged use of propanolol effectively decreases cardiac work in burned children. J Burn Care Rehabil 1997;18:223–7.

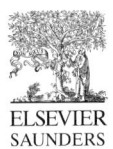

Management of Equine Poisoning and Envenomation

Gabriele A. Landolt, DVM, PhD

Department of Clinical Sciences, College of Veterinary Medicine and Biomedical Sciences, Colorado State University, 300 West Drake Road, Fort Collins, CO 80523, USA

Principles in the management of equine poisoning

Introduction

Acute poisoning commonly represents a diagnostic and therapeutic challenge facing the equine practitioner. Furthermore, although dealing with a single severely ill horse is demanding, toxicoses often involve multiple animals and can stimulate considerable emotion and publicity. When poisoning is suspected, every effort should be made to determine the potential source as well as the likelihood of exposure. Yet, although identification of the toxin is central for the protection of other animals and human beings from exposure, the emergency management of many toxicoses is primarily supportive. Regardless of the cause, the treatment and management of acutely ill animals have to be directed toward preserving the life of the animal. Therefore, the steps to successful treatment of equine poisoning are immediate emergency intervention, aggressive decontamination, supportive care, and careful monitoring of the animal.

Preventing further exposure

When first contacted by an owner concerning a potential poisoning, the client should be instructed to protect the animal from further exposure. In cases in which an environmental source is suspected, transport of the horse to the veterinary facility or relocation of the animal to a separate pen or stall can prevent further intoxication. It is also important to warn owners regarding hazards from human exposure to toxins (eg, on the horse's skin, in the environment) as well as to instruct them to use caution when handling the sick horse. In addition, the owner should be instructed to bring suspect

---

E-mail address: landoltg@colostate.edu

materials, their containers, or their labels with them to aid in the identification of the toxin. Most importantly, however, it is imperative that no time be wasted. The horse should be seen by the veterinarian as soon as possible.

Emergency intervention: stabilizing the acutely ill patient

The most critical aspect of emergency treatment is to ensure adequate function of vital organs to buy time for detoxification to occur and for specific antidotes to have their pharmacologic action. When multiple horses are involved, a triage system may be necessary. Emergency management may include establishment of a patent airway and provision of ventilatory and circulatory support as well as control of neurologic complications.

Maintenance of respiration

Inadequate ventilation caused by reduced respiratory effort or airway obstruction may require the provision of supplemental oxygen, a tracheotomy, or intubation with or without positive-pressure ventilation. If possible, arterial blood gas analysis should be undertaken in animals with dyspnea, hypoventilation, or hyperventilation or when metabolic acid-base disturbances are suspected. In comatose or anesthetized horses, a patent airway can be established using a cuffed endotracheal tube [1]. Mechanical forced ventilation may be necessary for horses with paralysis or severe central nervous depression or when general anesthesia is required to control seizures. Unfortunately, positive-pressure ventilatory support requires ventilator or anesthetic equipment that may not be available to the equine practitioner.

Maintenance of cardiovascular function

Normal cardiovascular function requires the presence of an adequate circulating volume, cardiac function, tissue perfusion, and acid-base and electrolyte balance. If shock or hypotension is present, intravenous fluids, such as balanced electrolyte solutions (eg, lactated Ringer's solution) or normal saline, are indicated. It is important to supply a sufficient quantity of fluids to replace deficits from previous losses (eg, hypersalivation, excessive sweating). Moreover, daily maintenance fluid requirements and ongoing losses (eg, diarrhea, polyuria) must be taken into account. A general guideline for maintenance fluid requirements is 50 to 80 mL/kg/d. Response to fluid administration (eg, changes in packed cell volume [PCV], total protein concentration, urine output, central venous pressure [CVP]) should be monitored closely during therapy to avoid fluid overload and help adjust flow rate. If hypovolemia is caused by loss of blood or plasma volume, a whole-blood or plasma transfusion may be indicated. The necessary volume of whole blood for a severely anemic horse can only be estimated. As a general rule, 10 to 20 mL/kg of body weight can be used to calculate blood replacement in clinically anemic animals (eg, PCV <12%–20%, hypovolemia, dyspnea).

Cardiac dysrhythmias (eg, bradycardia, tachycardia, arrhythmia) may manifest clinically as depression, weakness, ataxia, dyspnea, seizures, and death. In horses, possible agents that can be associated with life-threatening cardiac abnormalities include organophosphate and carbamate insecticides, Japanese yew, *Oleander* sp, foxglove, *Rhododendron* sp, and ionophore antibiotics (eg, monensin) [2,3].

If bradycardia is caused by organophosphate or carbamate toxicity, atropine sulfate should be administered. In horses, the recommended dose of atropine is 0.02–0.10 mg/kg of body weight. One fourth of this initial dose can be given intravenously, and the remaining volume should then be given intramuscularly or subcutaneously [4]. Atropine administration can be repeated if clinical signs reappear; however, caution should be exercised to avoid overdoses. Side effects of atropine include diminished respiratory, salivary, and gastrointestinal secretion as well as reduced intestinal motility and ileus (up to 9 hours after a single injection of atropine) [2].

The treatment of cardiac arrhythmias depends on the suspected etiology, the severity of the animal's clinical signs, and the electrocardiographic abnormalities detected [5,6]. In general, however, arrhythmias associated with poisoning should not be treated with antiarrhythmic drugs as a first-line approach [7]. Most antiarrhythmic agents have the potential to be proarrhythmic and negatively inotropic; thus, indiscriminate use of these agents in horses with intoxications is inadvisable. In addition, some antiarrhythmic drugs have been found to act synergistically with certain toxins (eg, digitalis glycosides, monensin) [8] and should thus not be used in acutely affected horses. The guiding principle in the management of cardiac arrhythmias in poisoned horses is to correct factors precipitating or contributing to the arrhythmia (eg, acidosis, hypokalemia, hypomagnesemia, hypoxia) [9]. Once the underlying disorder is resolved, cardiac arrhythmias often disappear spontaneously.

Central nervous system support

In large animals, the control of central nervous system (CNS) disturbances (ie, depression, hyperactivity) is often challenging, because overly aggressive therapy can turn CNS depression into hyperactivity (and vice versa). Horses that are agitated, restless, uncontrollable, or seizing must be sedated to enable therapy and to prevent injury, however. Moreover, generalized seizures should be treated immediately, because sustained seizure activity can result in severe hyperthermia, metabolic acidosis, hypoxia, and neurologic injury [10,11].

In adult horses and foals, commonly used drugs for seizure management include benzodiazepines (diazepam, 0.5–1.5 mg/kg administered intravenously) and barbiturates (pentobarbital sodium, 2–20 mg/kg administered intravenously; phenobarbital, 5–15 mg/kg in saline administered intravenously over 30 minutes). Large repeated doses of benzodiazepines should be avoided because they can cause excessive CNS and respiratory depression

[9]. In horses with resistant seizures or when long-term therapy is desired, administration of intravenous barbiturates is preferred. If anesthetic equipment is available, inhalant anesthetics have been used successfully in the long-term management of CNS hyperactivity [1,12]. Horses with severe muscle fasciculation may benefit from central muscle relaxants, such as methocarbamol (5–25 mg/kg administered intravenously slowly) [1,7,10]. Phenothiazines (eg, acepromazine, chlorpromazine) have been reported to reduce the seizure threshold and are therefore best avoided in the treatment of animals with CNS hyperactivity [2,7,13].

The use of analeptics, such as doxapram, methetharimide, and pentylenetetrazol, is controversial because their actions are fairly short lived and it may prove difficult to stabilize the animal receiving these drugs. In addition, convulsions and rebound depression after withdrawal are unwanted side effects. The most commonly used respiratory stimulant is doxapram (5–10 mg/kg administered intravenously). The drug is considered to have a narrow margin of safety, and large doses may result in seizures. In people, other reported adverse effects include hypertension, arrhythmias, and dyspnea [2].

Control of body temperature

Hyperthermia often occurs in patients with persistent seizures and in horses that have been poisoned with chlorophenol compounds (eg, pentachlorophenol [PCP], used as a wood preservative) [3,7]. Hyperthermia should be treated aggressively with cool intravenous fluids and active cooling measures (eg, ice bags, cold-water or alcohol baths, fans, cold-water enemas), because prolonged hyperthermia can result in significant complications, such as rhabdomyolysis, acute renal failure, and disseminated intravascular coagulopathy (DIC) [14,15]. Antipyretic drugs are generally not indicated in toxicant-induced hyperthermia [2].

Hypothermia may occur during anesthesia, heavy sedation, or coma. When body temperature is abnormally low, the rate of metabolic function (including poison degradation) is slowed. Blankets and heat lamps may be helpful in maintaining body temperature.

Topical exposure: skin decontamination

For dermal exposure with lipophilic substances (eg, insecticides), the horse's skin and hair coat should be washed with a mild detergent (eg, liquid dish detergent) using large volumes of warm water. Bathing should be repeated until the chemical odor is reduced or completely eliminated. Oily topical drugs or creams should not be used because they may increase the absorption of lipophilic toxins [2]. If the animal has been exposed to a dry or powdered toxin, bathing should not be undertaken, because wetting the compound may increase its absorption. Instead, removal of the poison from the animal's skin and hair coat can be accomplished by brushing or vacuuming. Caution must be exercised during the decontamination process to prevent human exposure, however. Protective clothing, including gloves, protective eyewear, long-sleeved clothing, and plastic aprons, should be used.

Ingested toxins: gastrointestinal decontamination

Gastric lavage

Gastric lavage involves the passage of a large-bore nasogastric tube and the sequential administration and aspiration of liquid with the intent of removing toxic substances present in the stomach. The value of gastric lavage in the management of intoxication is controversial. Several studies performed in dogs failed to demonstrate substantial drug recovery rates, particularly if the lavage was delayed 60 minutes or more after toxin ingestion [16–18]. Moreover, clinical studies in human patients found no evidence that gastric lavage improved patient outcome [19,20]. Proponents of the technique have argued that gastric lavage was not appropriately performed (eg, not sufficiently long, insufficient fluid volume used) in many of these studies, however [21]. To date, the clinical effectiveness of gastric lavage has not been tested in horses. Although gastrointestinal transit time can vary with the quantity and type of food present in the stomach, gastric lavage is most likely only beneficial in animals that are presented shortly after toxin ingestion [22]. In addition, coarse toxic plant material may be difficult to recover even when using tubes with a large diameter. To perform gastric lavage adequately, large-bore nasogastric tubes and copious amounts of lavage fluid are required. Water is instilled and removed until the returning water is clear. Recovered fluid and debris should be saved and refrigerated for toxicologic testing. Gastric lavage is contraindicated in unconscious horses without endotracheal intubation.

Activated charcoal

Activated charcoal (AC) is probably the best and safest adsorbing agent available to the equine practitioner. AC adsorbs toxins in the gastrointestinal tract and decreases the extent of absorption of the poison, thereby reducing or preventing systemic toxicity. Charcoal is produced by burning of coconut shells, peat, coal, wood, or petroleum. The charcoal is subsequently activated by heating in air, steam, or carbon dioxide, which results in the production of a highly developed pore structure and small particle size. The surface area of medicinal-grade activated charcoal typically ranges from 950 to 2000 m^2/g. AC is highly adsorptive for a large number of drugs and toxins (including insecticides, herbicides, and strychnine) but is less effective at adsorbing metals and alcohols [23]. Attachment of compounds to AC is nonspecific, and the number of drug or toxin molecules that can be adsorbed varies, depending on the solubility and ionization of the compound, pore size, particle size, and surface area of the charcoal; presence of inorganic salts; and gastric contents [24,25]. The optimal dose of AC is unknown, but data derived from experimental studies in human beings indicate a dose-dependent relation, which favors larger doses [26,27]. The suggested dose in horses ranges from 1 to 3 g/kg of body weight [1]. Several formulations of AC are available to the equine practitioner. Although easier to handle, compressed charcoal tablets have been shown to be inferior in the rate and extent of adsorption compared with powdered charcoal dispensed in water [28,29]. Furthermore, some liquid formulations contain preservatives, sorbitol (added for its cathartic properties), sodium bicarbonate, and povidone, which can potentially alter the efficacy of adsorption [23].

For AC to be effective, it must come in direct contact with the poison; thus, it should be given as soon as possible after the ingestion of a poison. A delay in charcoal administration reduces its effectiveness [30]. AC is often administered in combination with a saline cathartic. Although there are some experimental data supporting the benefit of this practice [31,32], the concurrent administration of oily cathartics, such as mineral oil, should be avoided, because lipids can substantially diminish the absorptive capacity of AC [33]. AC is best mixed with a sufficient amount of water to produce a slurry and is then given by nasogastric tube. Multiple-dose treatment regimens have been recommended for toxins that are primarily eliminated through hepatic metabolism and biliary excretion. The multidose treatment protocol is believed to interrupt enterohepatic cycling of such toxins [7,10]. A second benefit of the multidose treatment regimen is believed to come from the potential binding of any drug or toxin that passively diffuses along a concentration gradient from the circulation back into the lumen of the gastrointestinal tract [34]. The repeated administration of AC is believed to maintain this concentration gradient so that the toxin passes continuously into the gut lumen (a process that is also known as "gastrointestinal dialysis") [35]. Although animal studies and trials in human volunteers have demonstrated that multiple-dose AC treatment reduces the elimination half-life and increases drug clearance of some drugs [36–38], most of the clinical data supporting it have been derived from anecdotal case reports. Nevertheless, the single- or multidose AC treatment is simple, inexpensive, and safe. Complications associated with AC administration are rare. Adverse effects reported were not related to the agent itself but were a consequence of aspiration or direct administration of charcoal into the lungs [39].

Kaolin-pectin and bismuth compounds

Kaolin-pectin (Kaopectate, 2–4 L per 450 kg of body weight administered orally) and bismuth compounds (eg, bismuth subsalicylate, 1–2 L per 450 kg of body weight administered orally) are demulcents and have weak adsorbent properties. Although these compounds may have some benefits in the therapy for poisoned animals, their adsorptive capacities generally are inferior to those of AC [33].

Saline cathartics

The primary rationale for the use of cathartics is based on the belief that these agents reduce absorption of a toxin by accelerating its clearance from the gastrointestinal tract. The proposed mechanisms of action of saline cathartics are the promotion of osmotic retention of fluid and the extraction of water from the intestinal vasculature. The resulting increase in volume of gastrointestinal contents triggers intestinal motility reflexes, which subsequently leads to the enhanced expulsion of the intraluminal contents. Because most toxins are rapidly absorbed in the upper gastrointestinal tract (duodenum and proximal jejunum), the use of saline cathartics is most likely of primary benefit in animals that are treated shortly after poison ingestion and have been exposed to a slowly absorbed toxin. Unfortunately, no clinical studies have been published that have investigated the ability of cathartics to improve the outcome of toxicoses.

In horses, commonly used saline cathartics include sodium sulfate (Glauber's salt, 1 g/kg of body weight dissolved in 4 L of warm water and administered orally) and magnesium sulfate (Epsom salts, 0.2–1 g/kg of body weight dissolved in 4 L of warm water and administered orally) [1]. Sodium sulfate is a more effective saline cathartic than magnesium sulfate. In addition, excessive doses of magnesium sulfate, particularly in the presence of renal impairment, can cause signs of magnesium toxicity (eg, muscle weakness, CNS depression), enteritis, and dehydration.

Oily cathartics

Mineral oil and other oily cathartics are often less effective than other measures, such as the use of AC, with regard to diminishing the absorption of the toxin. Administration of mineral oil is valuable for treatment of poisoning involving lipid-soluble toxicants (eg, aliphatic hydrocarbons), however. In contrast to vegetable oil, mineral oil is inert and unlikely to be absorbed [12]. The simultaneous administration of an anionic surface-acting agent that decreases the surface tension (eg, dioctyl sodium sulfosuccinate [DSS]) should be avoided, because emulsification of the oil may contribute to its absorption [1].

Whole-bowel irrigation

Whole-bowel irrigation is a newer method of gastrointestinal decontamination that is used in human beings. The treatment consists of the enteral administration of large volumes (1500–2000 mL/h in adults) of an osmotically balanced polyethylene glycol electrolyte solution (eg, GoLYTELY; Braintree Laboratories, Braintree, Massachusetts). Whole-bowel irrigation is primarily used to treat ingestions of substances not effectively adsorbed by AC (eg, metals). Because the concentration of polyethylene glycol and electrolytes causes no net absorption or secretion of ions in the gastrointestinal tract, no significant fluid or electrolyte imbalances occur [40]. Although studies in dogs and people have demonstrated significant benefits from whole-bowel irrigation (eg, increased total body clearance, improved binding of toxin to charcoal when used in combination with whole-bowel irrigation), the procedure is in all probability not feasible in adult horses [41–43].

Increasing elimination

The treatments aimed at increasing the removal of already absorbed poisons are directed at an increase of the enzymatic conversion of the toxin to a less toxic metabolite, an increase in the rates of excretion of the poison, or the direct removal of the toxin from the affected animal (eg, by hemodialysis).

Enzymatic conversion

Although drugs capable of enhancing the activities of microsomal and soluble enzymes in the liver (eg, phenobarbital) have been used with the goal of reducing residues of persistent xenobiotics in tissues, these agents take at least a couple of days to increase enzymatic activity significantly. Therefore, the use of enzyme-inducing agents is not indicated in the acutely poisoned animal [33].

Promoting excretion

Many absorbed toxins are excreted by means of the kidneys. Thus, increasing the rate of renal elimination of the poison represents another potential target in the treatment of equine poisoning. Because the concentration of a toxin filtered at the glomerulus increases as water is reabsorbed during passage through the nephron, the resulting concentration gradient favors its absorption back into circulation. Forced diuresis enhances poison elimination by reducing its concentration (through dilution) in the filtrate, thus eliminating the gradient for reabsorption. Furthermore, increasing the filtrate's flow rate results in a reduction in the time spent in the tubule. Reabsorption can be further reduced by "trapping" the poison in the urine ("ion trapping") through manipulation of the urine pH. Ion trapping is based on the principle that a molecule's rate of diffusion through the basal membrane is reduced when the molecule is in an ionized state [44]. Enhanced renal elimination can be achieved using fluid diuresis or diuretics and by altering the urine pH [1,10,12,33].

Crystalloid fluids or, alternatively, large volumes of oral fluids given at a rate high enough to result in urine production of at least 2 mL/kg/h can optimize glomerular filtration and enhance clearance of renally eliminated toxins [10]. Such high fluid rates have to be administered with caution to avoid fluid overload, however. Pulmonary and renal function should be thoroughly evaluated before initiation of therapy, and fluid administration rates must be monitored carefully (eg, PCV, total protein, urine production). If available, CVP measurement offers an objective assessment of right ventricular filling pressure. Because CVP increases significantly in recumbent horses (values of 20–30 cm H_2O are not uncommon) [45,46], however, the horse's body position has to be taken into account for interpretation of CVP measurements. In addition, a single measurement of CVP is often of little value. Trends are most important in assessment of the volume status and cardiac function of the horse [47].

The use of diuretics to enhance urinary excretion of toxicants requires adequate renal function and hydration of the affected animal. The most commonly used diuretics include furosemide and mannitol [1,33]. Furosemide (0.5–1 mg/kg administered intravenously as needed) is a particularly potent short-acting agent that works by blocking the $Na^+/K^+/2Cl^-$ cotransporter in the ascending limb of the loop of Henle (loop diuretic). To be effective, however, furosemide must gain access to the lumen of the renal tubules. Thus, furosemide may be of limited value in horses with reduced renal perfusion or impaired renal function. Mannitol (0.25–1 g/kg administered intravenously as a 20% solution and given over 15–20 minutes) increases renal blood flow and the glomerular filtration rate. Once filtered, the agent also acts as an osmotic diuretic, thereby decreasing urine solute concentration and increasing urine volume. These agents are potent diuretics, and monitoring of urinary flow and the horse's hydration status is essential.

Urine alkalinization (also commonly referred to as "alkaline diuresis") is a treatment regimen that increases toxin elimination by administration of intravenous sodium bicarbonate to produce urine with a pH of 7.5 or greater [44]. The rationale behind this technique is based on the fact that at physiologic pH, most compounds exist partly in an undissociated state. Because cell membranes are more permeable for lipid-soluble (uncharged) molecules, the diffusion rate from the renal tubular lumen back into the circulation is greater for nonionized molecules than for charged molecules. Because ionization of weak acids (eg, salicylates, barbiturates, fluorides) is increased in an alkaline environment, increasing the urine pH can potentially enhance their renal excretion. Experimental data have demonstrated that the impact of urine alkalinization depends on the extent and duration of the pH change [44]. This means that a urine pH of at least 7.5 must not only be achieved but maintained if renal excretion of the poison is to be enhanced substantially. In addition, the effectiveness of this therapy depends on the relative contribution of renal clearance to the total body clearance of the drug [44]. In human beings, urine alkalinization is primarily used in the treatment of salicylate poisoning and was found to be of value [48,49]. Potential complications of intravenous bicarbonate administration include alkalosis, hypokalemia, and hypocalcemia [44].

In contrast to urine alkalinization, urine acidification (pH 5.5–6.0) is used to increase elimination of weak bases (eg, strychnine) and is generally accomplished by administering ammonium chloride. Administration of ammonium chloride requires acid-base monitoring and is contraindicated in animals with renal or hepatic impairment [33].

Direct toxin removal

Although hemodialysis is now being used successfully in small animals, the personnel, expertise, costs, and equipment required make its use unrealistic in large animals. Peritoneal dialysis, although standard practice in small animal medicine, is a difficult and time-consuming technique in large animal practice. Dialysis is particularly suited in anuric or oliguric patients to remove small water-soluble toxins with low protein binding (eg, barbiturates, bromide, gentamicin, salicylates, theophylline) [10]. The procedure involves the use of a dialysate solution (balanced electrolyte solution and dextrose [1.5%–4.25%]) that is infused into the peritoneal cavity at a rate of 10 to 20 mL/kg. The toxins move along a concentration gradient from the circulation into the dialysate. From 30 to 60 minutes after infusion, the dialysate is withdrawn and fresh solution is infused [1,10,12].

Antidotal therapy

Antidotes are only available for a limited number of drugs and poisons and are best considered with individual toxicants, and thus not discussed in this article. In general, caution should be exercised when using antidotes, because many of these agents are themselves toxic.

Principles in the management of equine envenomation

In the United States, poisonous snakes are estimated to bite several hundred horses each year, with between 10% and 30% resulting in fatalities [50]. Rattlesnakes are responsible for most venomous snakebites and for almost all deaths. Rattlesnakes are members of the family of pit vipers (Crotalidae), which also includes the cottonmouths (water moccasins) and copperheads. Coral snakes, which are indigenous to the coastal areas of the southeastern and western states to Texas, account for less than 3% of envenomation in people [51].

The venoms of pit vipers and coral snakes are complex mixtures of predominantly proteinaceous and peptidyl toxins that produce local and systemic effects. Local effects include edema formation, hemorrhage, skin necrosis, and myonecrosis. Systemic effects may comprise pre- or postsynaptic neurotoxicity, myotoxicity, pro- and anticoagulant activities, hemolysis, thrombocytopenia, cardiotoxicity, renal toxicity, and hypotensive or (rarely) hypertensive effects [52,53]. The extent of systemic effects depends on the concentration of toxins injected, the site of the bite, and the rate at which these toxins diffuse into the circulation [54]. Some of the factors reported to influence the amount of toxin injected include the snake species involved, age of the snake, time since the snake's last meal, and seasonal influences related to changes in feeding patterns or physiologic responses, such as hibernation [51]. In addition, not all bites result in envenomation. For example, in pit vipers, up to 20% of bites do not result in envenomation [55]. Therefore, the severity of clinical signs may vary considerably among snakebite victims.

Nevertheless, snakebites with envenomation should be regarded as an emergency, because irreversible effects of the venom begin immediately after toxin injection. Rapid clinical evaluation and appropriate treatment are paramount. Owners should be advised to keep the horse calm and limit its activity. Any interference with the wound should be avoided. Because venom is almost immediately absorbed into the surrounding tissue, incision over the fang marks is of minimal to no value [3]. Tourniquets, ligatures, and compression bandages should not be used because they increase local tissue damage attributable to hypoxia. The use of alcohol to clean the wound is contraindicated because its vasodilatory effect may promote spread of the venom [55]. Although once popular, surgical intervention with fasciotomy for venomous snakebite should be reserved for selected rare cases and should never be performed prophylactically [56].

Emergency intervention: stabilizing the acutely ill patient

The most life-threatening acute manifestations of rattlesnake envenomation in horses are airway obstruction and hemolytic anemia [57]. Most fatalities in horses are not associated with the acute poisoning, however, but are attributable to the development of fatal or debilitating diseases subsequent to envenomation (eg, debilitating heart disease, laminitis, myopathy, hepatopathy) [55,57]. Therefore, thorough clinical assessment of the degree of envenomation and (if indicated) emergency treatment should always be followed by careful monitoring of the animal. Emergency intervention should follow the same principles as discussed previously (see section on management of equine poisoning), including the establishment of a patent airway as well as the careful evaluation and monitoring of cardiovascular and pulmonary function.

The most consistent clinical signs associated with snakebite in horses are acute swelling and edema at the bite site [57]. In horses, bites frequently occur on the face, and subsequent swelling of the muzzle and external nares may result in partial or complete occlusion of the nasal passages. Insertion of a rigid tube (eg, endotracheal tube, large-bore syringe case opened on both ends) into the nasal passage may prevent complete occlusion. A tracheotomy may be required in horses with severe pharyngeal or laryngeal swelling, however. An emergency tracheotomy tube may be made from a cuffed endotracheal tube that has been shortened to reduce dead space [3] (Fig. 1).

Horses that exhibit severe systemic signs of envenomation (eg, coagulopathy, hemolysis, cardiac abnormalities, colic) should be treated with intravenous fluids [57]. Fluid therapy ensures adequate hydration, improves renal perfusion, and provides cardiovascular support. Some animals may develop such profound anemia attributable to hemolysis, coagulopathy, and hemorrhagic diathesis that whole-blood transfusion may become necessary (eg, persistent reduction of the PCV over a period of 24–48 hours to 12% or less) [58].

Antivenin therapy

There is a surprising lack of information on the effectiveness of antivenin therapy in horses. In people, however, parenteral administration of horse- or

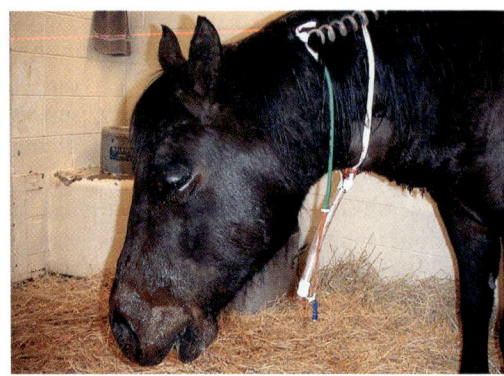

Fig. 1. Horse with head and neck swelling as a result of a rattlesnake envenomization. To ensure a patent airway, emergency tracheotomy was performed using a cuffed endotracheal tube.

sheep-derived antivenins constitutes the only scientifically validated treatment for moderate to severe snakebite envenomation [59,60]. Minimal envenomation has localized pain and swelling, normal vital signs and laboratory test results, and may not require antivenins [61]. There are two basic types of antivenins: monovalent and polyvalent. Monovalent antivenins, produced by immunization of an animal with one snake venom, contain specific antibodies against that particular venom. Polyvalent antivenins contain specific antibodies capable of neutralizing several venoms used in the immunization (often prepared against all relevant snakes in the particular area) [62] and can thus be administered without the need to identify the culprit snake.

Most available antivenins use immunoglobulins (eg, IgG) or their antigen-binding fragments (eg, Fab) to bind and inactivate the snake venom proteins. In the United States, two antivenins are marketed for the treatment of Crotalidae snake envenomation; an equine-derived serum globulin–based polyvalent antivenin (Fort Dodge Laboratories, Fort Dodge, Iowa) and an ovine-derived Fab polyvalent antivenin (CroFab; Altana, Melville, New York). Because IgG molecules themselves are antigenic, the use of serum globulin–based antivenins has been associated with the appearance of adverse effects [53,59,63], with their severity ranging from mild manifestations (eg, urticaria) to more severe complications (eg, anaphylactic shock, bronchospasm, hypotension) [59]. In contrast, Fab fragments are less immunogenic; thus, fewer adverse reactions have been reported with the Fab-based product in people [63,64]. At present time, only the equine IgG-based product is licensed for use in animals. In addition, the use of Fab-based products in veterinary medicine is limited because of their high cost [63].

Historically, antivenin often was given intramuscularly or subcutaneously; in some instances, it was also injected directly into the area of the bite. Yet, experimental studies have demonstrated that antivenin administered intravenously results in a more rapid, effective, and predictable response [65]. Unfortunately, optimal dose requirements of antivenins and duration of therapy have not been fully explored [66]. Ideally, the dose of antivenin should be based on measuring serial venom concentration and determination when free venom concentrations are undetectable [59]. This type of monitoring is not feasible in equine practice, however. In the absence of any definite data, dose recommendations vary substantially (10–50 mL [1–5 vials] administered intravenously) and depend on the severity of symptoms, time after bite, size of the snake, and size of the affected animal. A review of current human medical references shows a wide variation in the indications for and amount of antivenin to be used [56,66,67], and the recommended dose for the equine-derived Crotalidae Polyvalent Antivenin (Wyeth-Ayerst Laboratories, Philadelphia, Pennsylvania) ranges from 0 (mild envenomation) to 25 (life-threatening envenomation) vials for the initial treatment, followed by reassessment of the patient to determine if additional antivenin is needed [56,68,69]. In people, the total number of vials given has been reported to average 28.5 vials per patient [68,69].

Coral snake (elapid) venom contains primarily neurotoxic components, including a cholinesterase that produces the parasympathetic effects seen with elapid envenomation. Because of the lack of significant proteolytic enzyme activity, there is minimal to absent local swelling at the bite site [59]. An equine-origin elapid antivenin is available (Wyeth-Ayerst Laboratories).

Antibiotics, tetanus toxoid, and anti-inflammatory drugs

Although the incidence of infection after snakebite is poorly described, the prophylactic use of broad-spectrum antibiotics is a common practice in the treatment of snakebites [70]. In this regard, it is interesting to note that a number of studies of people with rattlesnake bites failed to document a significant incidence of infection subsequent to snake envenomation, despite the lack of antibiotic treatment [71,72]. Local tissue destruction and the high concentration of bacterial flora in the mouths of rattlesnakes (eg, *Pseudomonas aeruginosa*, *Clostridium* spp, *Staphylococcus* spp) [73] may justify the use of broad-spectrum antibiotic treatment for the prevention of wound infection and secondary complications, however. Once initiated, antibiotic therapy should be continued until the local swelling is resolved, fever has subsided, and the leukogram is normal [57]. In horses, tetanus antitoxin should always be administered. Nonsteroidal anti-inflammatory drugs can be given to control pain, swelling, and inflammation. Because they may enhance snake venom–induced thrombocytopenia, however, they should be used judiciously [3].

Corticosteroid administration

The use of corticosteroids in the treatment of snakebite is controversial [57,67]. Experimental and clinical studies have not been able to demonstrate a benefit of corticosteroid administration in cases of acute envenomation [57,74]. The consensus in human medicine is that their use is generally only indicated if allergic complications occur [67].

Summary

The goals for the management of toxicologic emergencies in the horse are directed toward immediate interventions to stabilize the animal's vital signs, prevention of continued exposure to the toxin, enhancement of the removal of the absorbed toxin, administration of an antivenin or antidote (if available), and initiation of supportive therapy as well as observation. In most cases, treatment of the animal must begin before an etiologic diagnosis is established; therefore, medical therapy should be focused on the clinical signs exhibited by the affected horse and should be based on sound veterinary medical principles.

References

[1] Bailey EM, Garland T. Management of toxicoses. In: Robinson NE, editor. Current therapy in equine medicine. Philadelphia: W.B. Saunders; 1992. p. 346–53.
[2] Beasley V. Diagnosis and management of toxicoses. In: Beasley V, editor. Veterinary toxicology. Ithaca (NY): International Veterinary Information Service; 1999. p. 1–28.
[3] Schmitz DG. Toxicologic problems. In: Reed SM, Bayly WM, editors. Equine internal medicine. Philadelphia: W.B. Saunders; 1998. p. 981–1042.
[4] Meerdink GL. Organophosphorus and carbamate insecticide poisoning in large animals. Vet Clin North Am Food Anim Pract 1989;5(2):375–89.
[5] Reef VB, McGuirk SM. Diseases of the cardiovascular system. In: Smith BP, editor. Large animal internal medicine. St. Louis (MO): Mosby; 1996. p. 507–49.
[6] Reimer JM, Reef VB, Sweeney RW. Ventricular arrhythmias in the horse: twenty-one cases (1984–1989). J Am Vet Med Assoc 1992;201(8):1237–43.
[7] Greene SL, Dargan PI, Jones AL. Acute poisoning: understanding 90% of cases in a nutshell. Postgrad Med 2005;81(954):204–16.
[8] Amend JF, Mallon FM, Wren WB, et al. Equine monensin toxicosis: some experimental clinicopathologic observations. Compend Cont Educ Pract Vet 1980;11(10):S173.
[9] Jones AL, Dargan PI. Churchill's pocket book of toxicology. London: Churchill Livingstone; 2001.
[10] Hackett T. Emergency approach to intoxications. Clin Tech Small Anim Pract 2000;15(2):82–7.
[11] Brown SA. Anticonvulsant therapy in small animals. Vet Clin North Am Small Anim Pract 1988;18(6):1197–216.
[12] Bailey EM. Emergency procedures in intoxications. Vet Clin North Am Small Anim Pract 1975;5(4):737–53.
[13] Markowitz JC, Brown RP. Seizures with neuroleptics and antidepressants. Gen Hosp Psychiatry 1987;9(1):135–41.
[14] Schrier RW, Henderson HS, Tisher CC. Nephropathy associated with heat stress and exercise. Ann Intern Med 1967;67(2):356–76.
[15] Vertel RM, Knochel JP. Acute renal failure due to heat injury. An analysis of ten cases associated with a high incidence of myoglobinuria. Am J Med 1967;43(3):435–51.

[16] Abdallah AH, Tye A. A comparison of the efficacy of emetic drugs and stomach lavage. Am J Dis Child 1967;113(5):571–5.
[17] Arnold FJ, Hodges JB, Barta RA. Evaluation of the efficacy of lavage and induced emesis in treatment of salicylate poisoning. Pediatrics 1959;23(2):286–301.
[18] Corby DG, Lisciandro RC, Lehman RH, et al. The efficiency of methods used to evacuate the stomach after acute ingestions. Pediatrics 1967;40(5):871–4.
[19] Comstock EG, Faulkner TP, Boisaubin EV, et al. Studies on the efficacy of gastric lavage as practiced in a large metropolitan hospital. Clin Toxicol 1981;18(5):581–97.
[20] Pond SM, Lewis-Driver DJ, Williams GM, et al. Gastric emptying in acute overdose: a prospective randomised controlled trial. Med J Aust 1995;163(7):345–9.
[21] Matthew H. Gastric aspiration and lavage. Clin Toxicol 1970;3(2):179–83.
[22] Meester WD. Emesis and lavage. Vet Hum Toxicol 1980;22(4):225–34.
[23] Neuvonen PJ, Olkkola KT. Oral activated charcoal in the treatment of intoxications. Role of single and repeated doses. Med Toxicol Adverse Drug Exp 1988;3(1):33–58.
[24] Andersen AH. Experimental studies on the pharmacology of activated charcoal. II. The effect of pH on the adsorption by charcoal from aqueous solutions. Acta Pharmacol 1947; 3(2):199–218.
[25] Watson WA. Factors influencing the clinical efficacy of activated charcoal. Drug Intell Clin Pharm 1987;21(2):160–6.
[26] Chin L, Picchioni AL, Bourn WM, et al. Optimal antidotal dose of activated charcoal. Toxicol Appl Pharmacol 1973;26(1):103–8.
[27] Olkkola KT. Effect of charcoal-drug ratio on antidotal efficacy of oral activated charcoal in man. Br J Clin Pharmacol 1985;19(9):767–73.
[28] Remmert HP, Olling M, Slob W, et al. Comparative antidotal efficacy of activated charcoal tablets, capsules and suspension in healthy volunteers. Eur J Clin Pharmacol 1990;39(5): 501–5.
[29] Tsuchiya T, Levy G. Drug absorption efficacy of commercial activated charcoal tablets in vitro and in man. J Pharm Sci 1972;61(4):624–5.
[30] Bond GR. The role of activated charcoal and gastric emptying in gastrointestinal decontamination: a state-of-the-art review. Ann Emerg Med 2002;39(3):273–86.
[31] Chin L, Picchioni AL, Gillespie T. Saline cathartics and saline cathartics plus activated charcoal as antidotal treatments. Clin Toxicol 1981;18(7):865–71.
[32] Galinsky RE, Levy G. Evaluation of activated charcoal-sodium sulfate combination for inhibition of acetaminophen absorption and repletion of inorganic sulfate. J Toxicol Clin Toxicol 1984;22(1):21–30.
[33] Beasley VR, Dorman DC. Management of toxicoses. Vet Clin North Am Small Anim Pract 1990;20(2):307–37.
[34] McKinnon RS, Desmond PV, Harman PJ. Studies on the mechanisms of action of activated charcoal on theophylline pharmacokinetics. J Pharm Pharmacol 1987;39(7): 522–5.
[35] Levy G. Gastrointestinal clearance of drugs with activated charcoal. N Engl J Med 1982; 307(11):676–8.
[36] Arimori K, Nakano M. The intestinal dialysis of intravenously administered phenytoin by oral activated charcoal in rats. J Pharmacobiodyn 1987;10(4):157–65.
[37] Chyka PA, Holley JE, Mandrell TD, et al. Correlation of drug pharmacokinetics and effectiveness of multiple-dose activated charcoal therapy. Ann Emerg Med 1995;25(3): 356–62.
[38] Neuvonen PJ, Elonen E. Effect of activated charcoal on absorption and elimination of phenobarbitone, carbamazepine and phenyl-butazone in man. Eur J Clin Pharmacol 1980;17(1): 51–7.
[39] Sato RL, Wong JJ, Sumida SM, et al. Adverse effects of superactivated charcoal administered to healthy volunteers. Hawaii Med J 2002;61(11):251–3.

[40] Davis GR, Santa Ana CA, Morawski SG, et al. Development of a lavage solution associated with minimal water and electrolyte absorption or secretion. Gastroenterol 1980;78(5):991–5.
[41] Arimori K, Deshimaru M, Furukawa E, et al. Adsorption of mexiletine onto activated charcoal in macrogol-electrolyte solution. Chem Pharm Bull 1993;41(4):766–8.
[42] Burkhart KK, Wuerz RC, Donovan JW. Whole-bowel irrigation as adjunctive treatment for sustained-release theophylline overdose. Ann Emerg Med 1992;21(11):1316–20.
[43] Mizutani T, Yamashita M, Okubo N, et al. Efficacy of whole bowel irrigation using solutions with or without adsorbent in the removal of paraquat in dogs. Hum Exp Toxicol 1992;11(6): 495–504.
[44] Proudfoot AT, Krenzelok EP, Vale JA. Position paper on urine alkalinization. J Toxicol Clin Toxicol 2004;42(1):1–26.
[45] Hall LW, Nigam JM. Measurement of central venous pressure in horses. Vet Rec 1975;97(4): 66–9.
[46] Klein L, Sherman J. Effects of preanesthetic medication, anesthesia, and position of recumbency on central venous pressure in horses. J Am Vet Med Assoc 1977;170(2):216–9.
[47] Bonagura JD, Reef VB. Cardiovascular diseases. In: Reed SM, Bayly WM, editors. Equine internal medicine. Philadelphia: W.B. Saunders; 2001. p. 290–370.
[48] Prescott LF, Balali-Mood M, Critchley JAJH, et al. Diuresis or urinary alkalinisation for salicylate poisoning? Br Med J 1982;285(6352):1383–6.
[49] Vree TB, Van Ewijk-Beneken Kolmer EW, Verwey-Van Wissen CP, et al. Effect of urinary pH on the pharmacokinetics of salicylic acid, with its glycine and glucuronide conjugates in human. Int J Clin Pharmacol Ther 1994;32(10):550–8.
[50] Burger CH, Van Gelder GA. Snakebite. In: Mansmann RA, McAllister ES, Pratt PW, editors. Equine medicine and surgery. Santa Barbara (CA): American Veterinary Publication Inc.; 1985. p. 215–7.
[51] Ellenhorn MJ, Barceloux DG. Medical toxicology. New York: Elsevier Science; 1988.
[52] White J. Overview of venomous snakes of the world. In: Dart R, editor. Medical toxicology. Philadelphia: Lippincott, Williams and Wilkins; 2004. p. 1543–59.
[53] Chippaux JP, Williams V, White J. Snake venom variability: methods of study results and interpretations. Toxicon 1991;29(11):1279–303.
[54] Kemparaju K, Girish KS. Snake venom hyaluronidase: a therapeutic target. Cell Biochem Funct 2006;24(1):7–12.
[55] Beasley V. Toxicants that affect peripheral circulation and/or may cause reduced lactation. In: Beasley V, editor. Veterinary toxicology. Ithaca (NY): International Veterinary Information Service; 1999. p. 1–16.
[56] Juckett G, Hancox JG. Venomous snakebites in the United States: management review and update. Am Fam Physician 2002;65(7):1367–74.
[57] Dickinson CE, Traub-Dargatz JL, Dargatz DA, et al. Rattlesnake venom poisoning in horses: 32 cases (1973–1993). J Am Vet Med Assoc 1996;208(11):1866–71.
[58] Moss DD. Diseases associated with blood loss or hemostatic dysfunction. In: Smith BP, editor. Large animal internal medicine. St. Louis (MO): Mosby; 1990. p. 1198–213.
[59] Lalloo DG, Theakston RDG. Snake antivenoms. J Toxicol Clin Toxicol 2003;41(3): 277–90.
[60] Theakston RDG, Warrell DA, Griffiths E. Report of a WHO workshop on the standardization and control of antivenoms. Toxicon 2003;41(5):541–57.
[61] Braun R, Krishel S. Environmental emergencies. Emerg Med Clin North Am 1997;15(2): 451–79.
[62] Raweerith R, Ratanabanangkoon K. Immunochemical and biochemical comparison of equine monovalent and polyvalent snake antivenoms. Toxicon 2005;45(3):369–75.
[63] Gwaltney-Brant SM, Rumbeiha WK. Newer antidotal therapies. Vet Clin North Am Small Anim Pract 2002;32(2):323–39.

[64] Seger D, Kahn S, Krenzelok EP. Treatment of US Crotalidae bites: comparison of serum and globulin-based polyvalent and antigen-binding fragment antivenins. Toxicol Rev 2005; 24(4):217–27.
[65] Gold BS, Barish RA. Venomous snakebites. Current concepts in diagnosis, treatment and management. Emerg Med Clin North Am 1992;10(2):249–67.
[66] Srimannarayana J, Dutta TK, Sahai A, et al. Rational use of anti-snake venom (ASV): trial of various regimens in hemotoxic snake envenomation. J Assoc Physicians India 2004;52: 788–93.
[67] Russell FE. Medical problems of snakebite. Snake venom poisoning. Great Neck (NY): Scholium International; 1983. p. 235–344.
[68] Holstege CP, Miller MB, Wermuth M, et al. Crotalid snake envenomation. Crit Care Clin 1997;13(4):889–921.
[69] Tanen DA, Ruha A-M, Graeme KA, et al. Epidemiology and hospital course of rattlesnake envenomation cared for at a tertiary referral center in central Arizona. Acad Emerg Med 2001;8(2):177–82.
[70] Kerrigan KR, Mertz BL, Nelson SJ, et al. Antibiotic prophylaxis for pit viper envenomation: prospective controlled trial. World J Surg 1997;21(4):372–3.
[71] LoVecchio F, Klemens J, Welch S, et al. Antibiotics after rattlesnake envenomation. J Emerg Med 2002;23(4):327–8.
[72] Clark RF, Selden BS, Furbee B. The incidence of wound infection following crotalid envenomation. J Emerg Med 1993;11(5):583–6.
[73] Goldstein EJ, Citron DM, Gonzalez H, et al. Bacteriology of rattlesnake venom and implications for therapy. J Infect Dis 1979;140(5):818–21.
[74] Cunningham ER, Sabboch MS, Smith RM, et al. Snakebite: role of corticosteroids as immediate therapy in an animal model. Am Surg 1979;45(12):757–9.

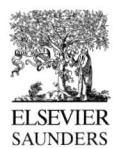

Ophthalmic Emergencies in Horses

Barbara Dallap Schaer, VMD

Department of Clinical Studies, George D. Widener Hospital for Large Animals, University of Pennsylvania School of Veterinary Medicine, New Bolton Center, 382 West Street Road, Kennett Square, PA 19348, USA

The equine eye is large and lies in a prominent and somewhat unprotected position in the equine skull. Given the horse's propensity to flight under circumstances of fright, orbital trauma is not uncommon in the emergency setting. Additionally, given the many varied occupations of horses, a highly visual species, in some rather harsh environments (eg, racetrack, hunt races, barrel racing), it is not unexpected that the horse incurs a moderate amount of corneal disease. It is therefore necessary for the equine emergency clinician to be fairly well versed in receiving and evaluating ophthalmic emergencies, provided that an ophthalmologist is not available consistently on an emergency basis. The most common emergencies encountered are orbital trauma, including eyelid lacerations, acute corneal trauma or laceration, and ulcerative keratitis or keratomycosis.

Orbital trauma

Initial evaluation

Orbital trauma can range in severity from minor impact associated with no globe damage and eyelid laceration only to fracture of the orbit and globe rupture. Blunt trauma of significant force may actually be more damaging to the horse from a visual standpoint, because intraocular structures are more likely to be disrupted. In rare cases, the impact can be severe enough to result in alterations of level of consciousness of the patient and likely represents traumatic brain injury. Initial assessment of the patient should therefore begin with evaluation of the entire patient, paying particular attention to the horse's demeanor and level of awareness. A complete physical examination should be performed, and as much information as possible should be obtained about the nature of the injury and the

E-mail address: bldallap@vet.upenn.edu

treatments the horse has received thus far. The time frame of the injury may be important with respect to the mental status of the patient, because alterations in awareness may lag hours behind the injury. Sedation must be used with caution in any patient in which brain injury is suspected, because severe exacerbation of symptoms may result.

During the initial evaluation, particular attention should be paid to facial, specifically orbital, symmetry (Fig. 1). Any degree of facial or orbital asymmetry could be associated with orbital fracture (Fig. 2) or possible globe rupture. The orbit should be carefully palpated for evidence of crepitus or instability to determine the index of suspicion of fracture or fractures. Abnormal globe positioning within the orbit can also be attributable to discontinuity of the orbital rim as a result of fracture [1]. The likelihood of involvement of the nasolacrimal duct should be evaluated as well as the continuity of the upper and lower eyelids. Based on this initial evaluation of external orbital structures, the need for additional diagnostics, such as radiography, dacryocystorhinography, or ultrasonography, can be determined.

Ocular examination

Complete ocular examination of both eyes allows the clinician to provide the owner with as much information as possible regarding the prognosis for vision. Evaluation of the noninjured eye cannot be overemphasized; owners are not always aware of visual deficits in their horses, and ocular trauma occasionally occurs secondary to a visual problem in the opposite eye.

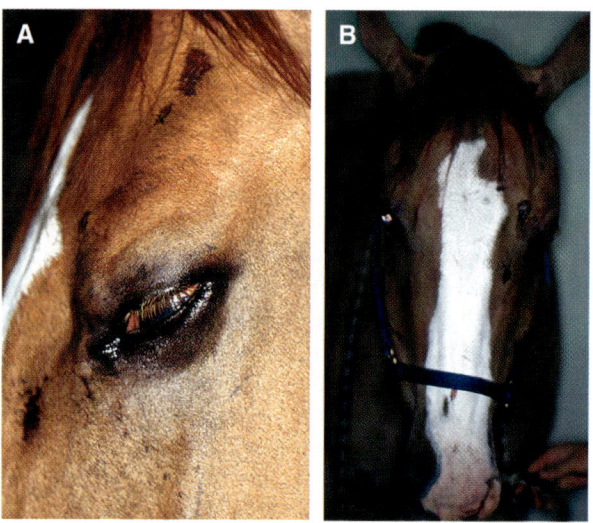

Fig. 1. Facial asymmetry caused by orbital trauma, with obvious periorbital soft tissue swelling: side (*A*) and front (*B*) views. (*Courtesy of* A. Komaromy, Dr Med Vet, PhD, Kennett Square, PA.)

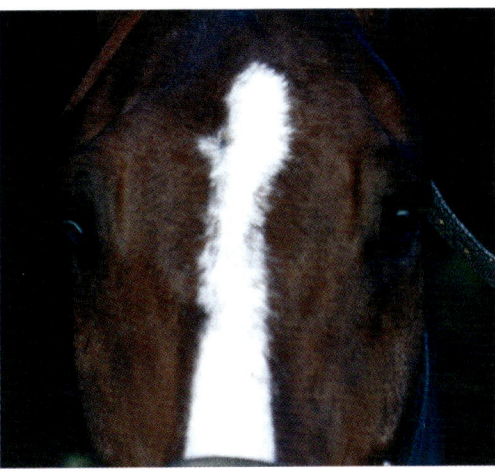

Fig. 2. Abnormal globe positioning of the left eye caused by previous orbital fracture. (*Courtesy of* A. Komaromy, Dr Med Vet, PhD, Kennett Square, PA, USA.)

Confirmation of the menace response can be accomplished by making cautious hand movements toward the injured eye, but putting the horse through a maze test to attempt to assess visual acuity is not recommended [2]. Eyelid function and continuity should also be evaluated, confirming proper lid closure and appropriate ability to protect the cornea. Critical first steps in assessing the prognosis for vision rely on evaluation of the direct pupillary light response (PLR), consensual PLR, and photophobic response ("dazzle"). Depending on the type, degree, and location of the trauma, it may be difficult to determine if a direct PLR exists, and a consensual PLR may be elicited only if an extremely bright light is used close to the injured eye. The presence of a consensual light response at least confirms the continuity of the visual pathway (retina and optic nerve) in the injured eye, meaning that a visual outcome may be possible. Similarly, a photophobic response or dazzle also establishes that the neural pathway is intact. The presence of persistent mydriasis (without the aid of a mydriatic) in the injured eye is indicative of an extremely poor outcome for vision [2].

Once initial evaluation of the menace and PLR responses are complete, the ocular structures should be examined in a systemic manner. The ophthalmic examination may be limited by the nature of the injury itself, and additional diagnostics, such as ultrasonography, may be needed. The horse should be adequately sedated or restrained for ocular examination, and motor nerve blocks are recommended to facilitate examination. Because of the strength of the orbiculus oculi in the horse, it is essential to perform motor nerve blocks before making any attempts to hold the eyelids open for ocular examination, particularly if the cornea is compromised [3]. An auriculopalpebral nerve block can be performed by injecting 2% mepivacaine at a dose of 3 to 4 mL at the base of the ear near the intersection with the edge of the zygomatic arch, which results in motor blockade predominantly of the upper eyelid but no desensitization of the lid or ocular structures [4]. Alternatively, the block can be performed at a more distal site, using 2% mepivacaine at a dose of 1 to 2 mL injected over the palpable palpebral branch of the auriculopalpebral nerve as it crosses the zygomatic arch. In some patients, desensitization of the lids may be useful, which can be accomplished by blocking the frontal nerve with local anesthetic (2% mepivicaine) at a dose of 2 to 3 mL placed subcutaneously over the palpable supraorbital foramen (dorsal to the medial canthus of the eye) [3]. Once the motor and sensory functions of the eyelids have been blocked and the horse is adequately restrained, the ocular structures can be safely examined.

Systematic attempts must be made to examine as many components of the eye as the injury allows. In many cases, the degree of chemosis and associated soft tissue swelling may make examination of the globe difficult. Corneal edema, hyphema, or hemorrhage into the posterior chamber may inhibit evaluation of the anterior chamber lens, the retina, or even the optic disk. In situations such as these, it may be advantageous to evaluate the globe ultrasonographically. Ultrasonographic evaluation can successfully identify rupture of the globe (Fig. 3), a detached retina (Fig. 4), lens luxation, or bony impingement of the orbit on the globe (Fig. 5). Such findings are crucial to the development of an immediate therapeutic plan. Caution must be taken to prevent absolutely any gel used for ultrasonographic examination from entering the palpebral fissure, however, and the patient must be appropriately sedated and restrained [3]. Proceeding to surgical exploration before ultrasonographic evaluation of the eye may result in unnecessary general anesthesia for an already potentially compromised patient. If additional diagnostics cannot be performed immediately, broad-spectrum

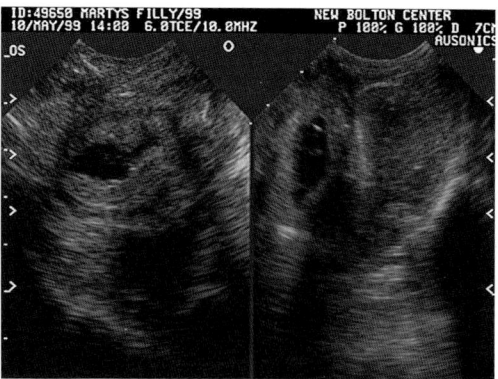

Fig. 3. Ultrasonography demonstrates rupture of the globe and complete disruption of intraocular structures.

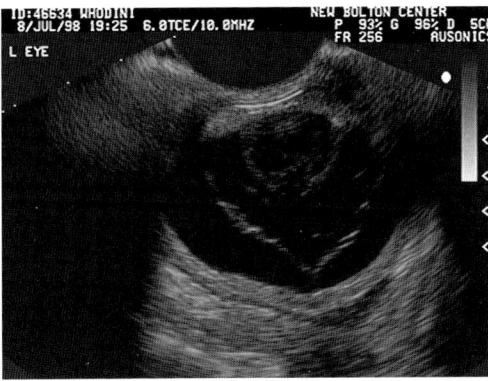

Fig. 4. Ultrasonography demonstrates retinal detachment, as evidenced by the V-shaped appearance of the retinal area of the globe.

antimicrobial therapy and anti-inflammatory therapy should be initiated until the patient can be re-evaluated or further diagnostics can be pursued.

The cornea should be carefully evaluated for any abrasions, punctures, or obvious lacerations. Any corneal laceration should be repaired surgically as an emergency under general anesthesia, preferably by a veterinary ophthalmologist with appropriate ophthalmic instrumentation. When advising owners or referring veterinarians in the initial management of corneal laceration or initiating treatment before referral to a veterinary ophthalmologist, it is imperative that only solutions be used for ophthalmic therapies [3]. No ointments should be placed in an eye with corneal laceration. To complete the corneal evaluation (see the sections on corneal laceration and corneal ulceration and ulcerative keratitis), adnexal structures should be closely examined for remnants of foreign bodies that may be responsible for corneal

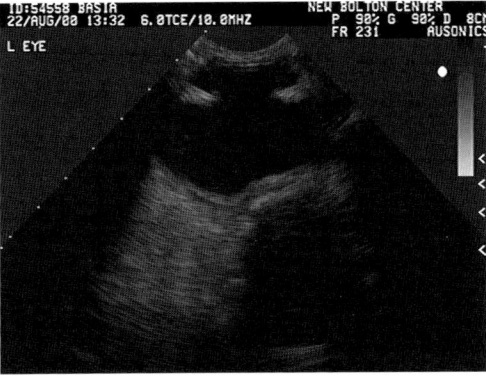

Fig. 5. Ultrasonography demonstrates bony impingement of the orbit on the globe, near the optic nerve, as a result of orbital trauma.

perforation or abrasion, the area should be cultured with a sterile moist swab, and fluorescein staining should be performed. After fluorescein staining, the eye should be closely evaluated under magnification (direct ophthalmoscope or slit-lamp biomicroscopy), possibly with the use of a cobalt blue filter, to evaluate the corneal surface meticulously for any defects or wound margins. If indicated, the cornea can be desensitized (0.5% proparacaine hydrochloride or 0.5% tetracaine hydrochloride) and corneal scraping can be performed (see the section on corneal ulceration and ulcerative keratitis). Any positive fluorescein findings as well as the degree of corneal edema should be carefully documented to serve as a baseline for progression of corneal disease. The Seidel test, performed by placing concentrated fluorescein (orange) on the corneal lesion (after topical anesthesia) and watching for aqueous streaming (green) under a cobalt blue filter, can be used to detect small corneal punctures or to characterize small full-thickness corneal lacerations [5].

The anterior chamber should be evaluated for flare, hyphema, and hypopyon. If the means are available, intraocular pressures (IOPs) can also be recorded using applanation tonometry (Tono-Pen; Oculab, Baltimore, Maryland), provided that they can be safely obtained. Reported normal values for IOP in the horse are reported to range from 17.1 to 29.6 mm Hg [6]. Both eyes should be evaluated, and there should be a difference less than 5 mm Hg between them [7]. Sedation may decrease the IOP in a horse by as much as 25% [8]. Digital tonometry may be inappropriate if severe compromise to the corneal integrity is evident. Assessment of the degree of inflation of the anterior chamber may be determined visually in such circumstances, using the noninjured eye for comparison. To complete the examination, direct ophthalmoscopy or slit-lamp biomicroscopy should be used to determine the lens position and thoroughly evaluate the fundus.

Orbital fractures

Fractures of the bones comprising the orbit are less common than other skull fractures but do occur as a result of sudden movement in a confined space or kick injury. The bony orbit is a combination of the temporal bone (zygomatic process) laterally, the frontal bone (including the zygomatic process) dorsally, the lacrimal bone medially just under the medial canthus, and the zygomatic bone ventrally [9]. Orbital fractures can be diagnosed radiographically, by digital assessment, or, if available, by MRI or CT. Fractures typically include some portion of the supraorbital process or zygomatic arch, or they may involve the area adjacent to the medial canthus [9]. Fractures of the frontal bone or zygomatic bone can extend axially or rostrally to involve the frontal or caudal maxillary sinus, respectively [10]. Significant damage to the lacrimal bone medially could result in damage to the nasolacrimal duct, and patency of the duct should be confirmed by flushing or dacryocystorhinography. Standard radiographic views for the diagnosis of an orbital fracture include lateral and dorsoventral projections as well as a dorsoventral oblique view projecting the affected side. Orbital fractures can be difficult to project radiographically, and a ventrodorsal projection of the affected side with the plate positioned on the horse's forehead may be the most useful view (Carole Johnson, personal communication, 1998) (Fig. 6).

The decision to repair the fracture surgically or to manage it conservatively should be based on other relevant factors, such as impingement on ocular structures (optic nerve or globe) or adnexal structures (supraorbital nerve or nasolacrimal duct). Alternatively, surgery may be elected to be performed for cosmetic reasons only, although definitive cosmetic improvement by surgical intervention is not necessarily guaranteed.

There are essentially two surgical techniques commonly used for repair of orbital fractures. Closed reduction under general anesthesia using digital retraction or bone hooks cautiously placed into the dorsal conjunctival fornix is often successful for treatment of fractures of the dorsal rim that are closed and relatively simple [10]. Open exploration and reduction are more useful for fractures that are severely comminuted, open, or more than 60 hours old [9,10]. Reduction of fractures of the lacrimal bone, zygomatic process of the frontal or temporal bone, and zygomatic bone may be better accomplished by open reduction [10]. Methods of stabilization include stainless-steel wire or polydioxanone suture. In situations in which the fragments interdigitate and stay in reduction, implants may not be necessary. If sinus involvement is also suspected based on surgical exploration or confirmation

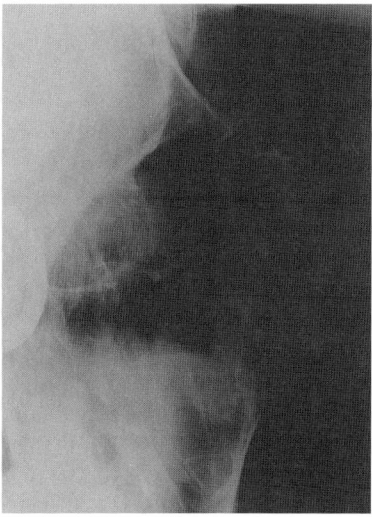

Fig. 6. Ventrodorsal oblique projection of the affected orbit after injury reveals comminution of the bony orbit.

by radiography, sinus lavage may be necessary at the time of surgery, with repeated irrigation after surgery.

Horses with open orbital fractures, including those fractures with no external wound but with communication confirmed by way of the frontal or caudal maxillary sinus, should be treated with systemic antimicrobial therapy and anti-inflammatories. Closed fractures that are managed conservatively can be treated with anti-inflammatories and antimicrobial therapy at the discretion of the clinician or based on the extent of other ocular injuries. Possible complications in horses with surgical treatment of orbital fractures include temporary postoperative depression of the palpebral reflex, perhaps attributable to inflammation or manipulation of the auriculopalpebral nerve, and traumatic uveitis [10]. In a small series evaluating horses with periorbital fractures, more than half had some degree of ocular injury, ranging from corneal ulceration to exophthalmus. A complete ophthalmic examination at admission and repeated ocular evaluations after surgery are definitively necessary in the treatment of horses with orbital fractures.

Eyelid lacerations

Eyelid lacerations are a relatively common injury, possibly attributable to the horse's rapid head movement response when startled or threatened. Lacerations of the upper lid are more common and more significant, because the upper lid is primarily responsible for tear film distribution and prevention of exposure keratitis. Eyelid lacerations should be promptly and surgically repaired. Do not remove any supposedly unneeded eyelid tissue or flap. The main goal of eyelid laceration repair is to maintain the absolute integrity of the entire lid margin as best as possible. Inappropriate eyelid laceration repair, failure to treat, overly aggressive eyelid debridement, or removal of the lid margin could result in a chronically painful eye with persistent exposure keratitis [11]. A complete ocular examination must also be completed, including fluoroscein staining, to determine if any corneal injury has occurred.

Simple lacerations can often be repaired in the standing horse under sedation and local anesthesia. An auriculopalpebral nerve block can be performed to block movement of the eyelid in addition to branches of the dorsal buccal nerve along the facial crest to reduce movement of the lower lid [4]. Sensory blockade of the central portion of the upper lid can be achieved by performing a frontal (supraorbital) nerve block. The needle is placed near the supraorbital foramen, and local anesthetic (2% mepivicaine) at a dose of 2 to 3 mL is injected [12]. If complete desensitization of the upper lid is needed, the lateral portion of the lid can be desensitized by performing a lacrimal nerve block. This is accomplished by positioning the needle subcutaneously just dorsal to the lateral canthus and directing it medially across the dorsal orbital rim during injection [12]. The medial canthus is blocked by placing a needle along the bony notch on the dorsal rim of the orbit (toward the medial canthus) and injecting a local anesthetic (2% mepivicaine) at a dose of 2 to 3 mL (infratrochlear nerve block) [12]. This block also produces desensitization of the medial portion of the lower lid. To obtain desensitization of the remainder of the lower lid, a zygomatic nerve block is necessary. This block is performed by injecting local anesthetic (3–5 mL, 2% mepivicaine) along the ventral and lateral aspect of the bony orbit, near the juncture where the orbit begins to curve upward [12].

More complicated eyelid lacerations, an uncooperative patient, or injuries involving surgical treatment of the cornea are all indications for repair under general anesthesia. Lavage of the wound to remove gross debris and foreign material with a pH-balanced polyionic electrolyte solution can be followed by aseptic preparation of the eyelid for surgical intervention. A 10% povidone-iodine solution should be used to prepare periocular tissues surgically; scrub preparation or chlorhexidine should never be used for surgical preparation for any surgery near the eye [3]. The wound itself can be prepared using a 5% povidone-iodine solution. During the surgical preparation, the cornea should be kept continually moist with an ophthalmic wetting solution to prevent corneal injury. Application of topical anesthesia to the cornea may facilitate repair even if the horse is under general anesthesia [3].

During eyelid laceration repair, minimal debridement of the eyelid margin is critical. Aggressive removal of what seems to be devitalized tissue may result in an undesirable outcome. Eyelids are extremely well vascularized, and many apparently "devitalized" portions of the lid survive after repair. Repair is typically performed in two layers and is initiated at the lid margin to ensure proper lid alignment. The first suture is commonly a figure-of-eight suture or a cruciate or mattress suture placed to align the lid margin perfectly (Fig. 7) [3]. This suture can be preplaced, and the deep layer can be closed by placing a continuous pattern of 5-0 or 6-0 absorbable suture in the tarsal plate, making sure that sutures do not penetrate the conjunctiva. Skin closure can be completed (4-0 to 6-0 nonabsorbable suture) in a simple interrupted pattern starting from the lid margin [5]. Care must be taken to ensure that no sutures are able to contact the cornea; trapping the preceding long suture tail in following knots may be a helpful tip to prevent this from happening.

Horses undergoing surgical repair for eyelid laceration should receive perioperative antimicrobial therapy, anti-inflammatories, and systemic tetanus prophylaxis. If the cornea is involved in the injury, a subpalpebral lavage (SPL) catheter should be placed while the horse is under general anesthesia or sedated with the lid blocked. Ophthalmic medications should be continued based on the severity and progression of corneal disease.

Corneal laceration

If at all possible, horses with a full-thickness corneal laceration should be referred to a veterinary ophthalmologist. Prompt surgical intervention by an ophthalmic surgeon with appropriate ophthalmologic surgical equipment can provide the horse and owner with the best chance for a favorable

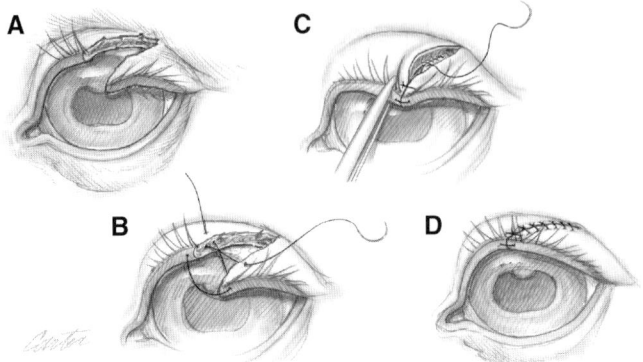

Fig. 7. Step-by-step depiction of eyelid laceration repair. (*A*) Wound is cleansed and minimally debrided. (*B*) Figure-of-eight suture at the eyelid margin allows alignment of the eyelid margin, which is critical to an effective repair. (*C*) Two-layer closure is performed if possible. The deep layer should start at the eyelid margin as well and proceed distally from it. (*D*) Simple interrupted skin sutures finish the closure. (*From* Capaldo F, Komáromy AM. Ophthalmic emergency. Current Techniques in Equine Practice 2006;5:135; with permission.)

outcome. A poor outcome for vision is associated with extensive ocular infection as a result of corneal penetration, extensive hyphema (>50%), disruption of intraocular contents, lacerations greater than 15 mm, or lacerations with scleral involvement [3,13,14]. Enucleation is probably the best option in horses with an extremely poor outcome for vision.

Corneal lacerations that have a fair chance for visual outcome often have a relatively formed anterior chamber, a small amount of hemorrhage in the eye, minimal corneal edema and associated infection or inflammation, and a relatively small amount of iris prolapse. Prompt and appropriate surgical intervention is necessary if vision is to be saved, and it must be emphasized that no ointments should be placed in an eye suspected to have a full-thickness corneal laceration. This is an important point to stress to owners, trainers, and referring veterinarians. Typically, corneal lacerations amenable to repair have readily recognizable ocular architecture, with a corneal defect plugged with iris or fibrin, decreased IOP, positive fluorescein at the laceration margins, and a positive dazzle and PLR (direct and consensual).

Full-thickness lacerations with iris prolapse or wound separation greater than 2 mm must be surgically repaired under general anesthesia [3]. If a veterinary ophthalmologist is not available, verbal consultation or review of a surgical ophthalmic textbook is suggested. Before surgery, the horse should receive systemic broad-spectrum antimicrobials and anti-inflammatories. Ophthalmic medications can be considered but only if the risk of exacerbation of the injury is deemed to be minimal [2,13,14]. It has been recommended that ketamine hydrochloride be avoided as part of the anesthetic protocol [3], and attempts should be made to protect the eye during induction. Neuromuscular blockade or local motor and sensory blocks may greatly facilitate successful completion of the procedure. The eyelashes can be clipped to facilitate aseptic preparation. The eye can be prepared for surgery using a 1:50 dilution of povidone-iodine (not scrub), rinsing the corneal and conjunctival fornix until sterile cotton applicators inserted in the surrounding conjunctiva appear clean. It is critical the corneal surface be kept moist until the surgery begins and throughout the entire surgical procedure.

Particularly in older lacerations, a devitalized or severely contaminated iris can be carefully trimmed to facilitate replacement posteriorly and minimize further contamination of the intraocular structures. Cautery may be useful in controlling hemorrhage after iridectomy [13]. The corneal laceration can be repaired using 6-0 to 8-0 ophthalmic polygalactin 910 in a simple interrupted or, occasionally, mattress pattern [2,3,13,14]. Sutures should be placed 1 to 2 mm apart deep into stromal tissue (three-quarters depth recommended) but not penetrating full thickness [3]. It is optimal to have entry and exit points of the suture positioned perpendicular to the corneal surface [3]. Jagged or irregular lacerations can be addressed by strategically placing sutures to reduce the gaping cornea to opposed linear wounds, which can then be routinely repaired [2,14]. It may be necessary to use to a cyclodialysis spatula or iris repository to retract the iris while suturing the cornea to prevent entrapment in the closure [14]. Throughout repair, lavage of the anterior chamber or inflation of the chamber may be necessary to remove hemorrhage and facilitate closure. After successful corneal repair, reinflation of the anterior chamber may be accomplished using a sterile balanced saline solution or lactated Ringer's solution or by use of viscoelastic materials, such as sodium hyaluronate. A conjunctival flap may be performed at the discretion of the surgeon to add additional support to the repair. Installation of an SPL system is recommended while the horse is under general anesthesia to facilitate medical management of the eye after surgery.

Postoperative management typically consists of systemic broad-spectrum antimicrobial therapy and anti-inflammatory therapy as well as topical 1% atropine and antimicrobial and antifungal therapy. Administration of serum or ethylenediaminetetraacetic acid (EDTA) may also be useful. Dosing frequency of ophthalmic medications may be as often as every 1 to 2 hours initially but should be modified based on the clinical progression of the eye. Repeat ophthalmic evaluation of the eye daily (or twice daily) is necessary to assess the response to surgical intervention and guide postoperative management. Secondary uveitis and endophthalmitis are common sequelae to surgically repaired corneal lacerations [3]. Worsening of the appearance of the corneal wound or wound dehiscence would be an indication for repeating corneal culture and sensitivity testing, because the organisms involved or antibiotic resistance of those organisms may have changed.

Partial-thickness lacerations or abrasions can be treated similar to corneal ulceration (see the section on corneal ulceration and ulcerative keratitis). A deep partial-thickness corneal flap still attached to the cornea can be repaired in a manner similar to a corneal laceration [2,3], and a thin flap with minimal edema can be reattached with tissue adhesive [2].

Corneal ulceration and ulcerative keratitis

Corneal abrasion and ulcerative keratitis are common reasons for emergency referral for ophthalmic evaluation. Again, the positioning of the equine eye, in combination with a horse's disposition, predisposes the horse to corneal injury. This, in combination with the horse's environment, and perhaps with the eye's inflammatory response to corneal injury, makes ulcerative keratitis a significant problem. Horses with corneal ulceration may be presented with epiphora, blepharospasm, photophobia, ocular discharge, or corneal edema.

Corneal ulceration is defined as a loss of corneal epithelium and exposure of the underlying corneal stroma. Appropriate assessment, in combination with timely and aggressive intervention, can prevent corneal ulceration from progressing into a vision-threatening condition. Cornea ulcers can be classified according to their severity and are often described as a superficial, moderate, or deep stromal ulcer; a descemetocele; or having a stromal abscess. Multiple differential diagnoses must be considered for ulcerative keratitis, including bacterial keratitis, fungal keratitis, or a combination of both, as well as iris prolapse, and even corneal laceration or perforation. Additionally, several inflammatory conditions must be considered, including eosinophilic keratitis, corneal degeneration, and intraocular disease [15]. Presentation of a horse for emergency evaluation of an ulcer or progressing ulcerative keratitis necessitates a thorough ophthalmic examination. A thorough history must be taken from the owner or referring veterinarian regarding the duration of the ulcerative disease; treatments attempted, including frequency; and any pending or final results of microbiologic culture and sensitivity testing. In addition to referring to the previous section on ocular examination, the following points can be made with respect to evaluating such a patient.

Tear production and corneal sensitivity should be evaluated, obviously before performing any blocks that facilitate ocular examination. Lid function should be assessed and critical examination of the adnexal structures should be performed to rule out additional ongoing problems that may be inciting causes of the disease process or responsible for exacerbation of clinical signs [3,15]. Eyelid akinesia should be established to complete the ocular examination. A rapid worsening of clinical signs, failure to respond appropriately to treatment, obvious stromal involvement, or keratomalacia is a sign of infectious keratitis, and microbiologic culture and sensitivity testing should be performed. This can be accomplished with the use of a sterile moist cotton swab before desensitization of the cornea (many topical ophthalmic anesthetics contain antimicrobials). A thorough examination under magnification should follow, paying particular attention to structures adjacent to the ulcerated area for a possible foreign body [3]. Fluorescein staining should follow, with careful documentation of the exact positioning of the ulcer, ulcer depth, degree of vascularization, and extent of edema. Assessment of anterior chamber and pupil size should also be carefully recorded. Particular attention should be paid to the character of the cornea affected, with the concern being detection of possible keratomalacia. Melting ulcers, commonly caused by *Pseudomonas* species or β-hemolytic *Streptococcus equi* (subspecies *zooepidemicus* or *equi*) [16], can result in rapid progression to keratolysis and perforation. Identification of an ulcer as melting is essential to direct aggressive medical therapy or suggest surgical intervention. In obviously infected or complicated ulcerative keratitis cases, a topical anesthetic should be applied and corneal scraping should be performed for cytologic evaluation. Surface debris should be removed before performing corneal scraping for cytologic evaluation to obtain a more diagnostic sample, and several slides should be made. Slides can then be Gram stained and evaluated for the presence of bacteria and fungi, because these preparations direct initial antimicrobial or antifungal therapy. Gram-negative rods may suggest the presence of *Pseudomonas* species, and if supported by clinical findings, anticollagenase therapy should be initiated. Gram-positive cocci may be commonly associated with *Staphylococcus* or *Streptococcus* species [5]. If possible, slides should be submitted to a clinical pathologist for further evaluation.

Treatment of ulcerative keratitis is directed at controlling infection and inflammation and promoting corneal healing while preventing secondary complications that may threaten visual outcome. Successful management may involve medical therapy only or may comprise a combination of surgical and medical therapies. Corneal ulcers that fail to heal in a relatively short time (<7 days) require more aggressive treatment, including repeat microbiologic culture and sensitivity testing, assessment for fungal elements, inspection for a corneal foreign body, increased protease control, or possible surgical intervention.

Medical management should include placement of an SPL catheter system to facilitate frequent medication administration with minimal risk for additional corneal trauma. An auriculopalpebral (motor) nerve block, frontal nerve block (sensory), and topical anesthetic applied to the cornea as well as sedation and adequate restraint permit safe placement of the SPL system. Single-hole catheters designed for SPL use are commercially available (Subpalpebral eye lavage kit, 12-gauge trocar, 36-in catheter; catalog no. 6612; Mila International, Florence, Kentucky); alternatively, polyethylene tubing with a handmade foot plate can be used [17]. SPL systems are more commonly placed in the most dorsal portion of the upper lid, making sure that the catheter rests in the conjunctival fornix and has no contact with the cornea [15]. The SPL catheter should be snuggly secured to the horse's head using a combination of tape and suture, ensuring that its position with respect to the conjunctival fornix is maintained. Alternatively, the SPL system can be placed in the lower lid (inferomedial placement), resting between the lower eyelid and the nictitans [18]. The catheter is usually fitted with an injection cap and device to protect the tubing-cap interface (eg, tongue depressor, tuberculin syringe). The tubing is typically fed through braids at the horse's forelock and mane to protect the tubing and facilitate treatment. Complications associated with SPL catheter therapy include catheter-associated mechanical ulceration caused by loosening of the system or suboptimal placement, medication leakage, catheter breakage, and lid swelling [17–19].

Antimicrobial selection should be based on examination of Gram-stained slides initially and can be modified on obtaining microbial culture and sensitivity testing results. Topical broad-spectrum antimicrobials, such as chloramphenicol or triple-antibiotic preparations (bacitracin-neomycin-polymyxin B) can be used in uncomplicated corneal ulcers [5], but more complicated ulcers or those failing to respond to therapy should be placed on more aggressive antimicrobials based on cytologic findings. Common isolates in more complicated ulcerative keratitis patients include *Streptococcus*, *Staphylococcus*, or *Pseudomonas* species. *Pseudomonas*-associated keratitis has long been associated with significant keratomalacia or melting corneal ulcers; therefore, aggressive antiprotease therapy, such as serum, EDTA, or acetylcysteine, should be a component of therapy in cases in which *Pseudomonas* species are identified or suspected. Control of inflammation systemically with flunixin meglumine as well as administration of 1% atropine is also recommended. β-Hemolytic streptococcal infection has also been associated with significant keratomalacia and the development of severe corneal disease, making it necessary to take a similar approach in cases in which cytologic evidence supports its presence [16]. In previous studies evaluating sensitivity in equine corneal disease, *Pseudomonas* species have been reported to be sensitive to polymyxin B [20], gentamicin [20,21], tobramycin [21], and fluoroquinolones [22]. *Pseudomonas* species seem particularly adept at developing resistance, and failure to respond to antipseudomonal antibiotics indicates that repeat culture and sensitivity testing should be performed. Evidence exists for alterations in antibiotic resistance over time, with a Florida study reporting *S equi* subspecies *zooepidemicus* becoming more resistant to gentamicin and *Pseudomonas aeruginosa* becoming more resistant to gentamicin and tobramycin over a 10-year period [23]. Because of the emergence of topical fluoroquinolone resistance in *P aeruginosa* infections in human keratitis, concerns about unjustified use of such topical treatments in horses exist [22], and therapy with higher generation fluoroquinolones (eg, moxifloxacin, gatifloxacin) has been suggested when indicated by culture [15].

Control of protease activity may be critical for successful treatment of aggressive ulcerative keratitis. Options include autologous serum, EDTA, *N*-acetylcysteine, and heparin [3,5,15]. Studies indicate that matrix metalloproteinase (MMP) levels in tear film are increased in horses with ulcerative keratitis and that levels correspondingly decrease with corneal improvement [24]. Serum is readily available and inexpensive, and it has activity against MMPs and serine proteases [15].

Systemic anti-inflammatories (flunixin meglumine, 1.1 mg/kg administered intravenously or orally twice daily) may be critical in controlling inflammation and maintaining the overall comfort of the horse, possibly preventing additional systemic complications. Topically applied 1% atropine is used as a mydriatic and for prevention of ciliary body spasm. Atropine should be applied until mydriasis is achieved [15], but horses should be monitored carefully for systemic atropinization and gastrointestinal ileus or discomfort [25].

Fungal keratitis seems to have become geographically more widespread in recent years. Clinically, fungal keratitis may appear as fluffy fungal plaques of varying color (gray, white, or yellow) and depths within the corneal stroma [15]. Reports for visual outcome vary in the literature from 53% [26] to 92% [27], but the presence of fungal elements in ulcerative keratitis is always reason for concern and indicative of the need for aggressive intervention. Fungal isolates associated with keratomycosis reported in the literature vary, but *Aspergillus* and *Fusarium* are overrepresented [15]. Natamycin is the only commercially available ophthalmic antifungal preparation in the United States and has been reported to be relatively effective against *Aspergillus* and *Fusarium* species [28]. Other available topical antifungals include itraconazole, miconazole, and ketoconazole [15,28]. Combined broad-spectrum antimicrobial therapy is also indicated for the treatment of keratomycosis. A recent study touting the efficacy of equine corneal penetration of voriconazole has led to an increase in its use for equine keratomycosis, but evidence of its efficacy in clinical trials is not yet reported [29].

Failure of the equine eye with ulcerative keratitis to respond to aggressive medical therapy indicates the need for critical reassessment, including repeat cytologic evaluation or surgical intervention. Indications for surgery, possibly conjunctival flap placement or amniotic membrane transplantation, may include middle to deep stromal ulcer depth, presence of a descemetocele, or continued progressive keratomalacia [30]. Other indications for surgery may include a corneal stromal abscess or progressive keratomycosis with a furrow surrounding the fungal lesion. Corneal stromal abscesses may appear as a focal stromal opacity associated with uveitis and often have a negative fluorescein result. In the face of a poor response to medical therapy, such conditions may improve with penetrating keratoplasty (PK) or posterior lamellar keratoplasty (PLK). Consultation of a veterinary ophthalmologist is strongly recommended for surgical intervention and is essential for PK or PLK.

Acute blindness

Occasionally, a horse with acute blindness is presented as an emergency in an equine referral setting. The most common cause of acute blindness, without any preceding observed ocular disease, is blunt trauma resulting in traumatic optic neuropathy. The severity of the condition may range from significant visual impairment to complete blindness. The globe itself is usually not injured, but the horse is often presented with obvious visual deficits and widely dilated pupils. The proposed mechanism is neuropraxia or significant trauma to the optic nerve or chiasm [31]. Clinically, the initial ophthalmic examination may reveal no significant ocular lesion in the face of a negative menace response, negative photophobic response, and no PLR. Later (several weeks) ophthalmic examinations may reveal optic nerve pallor and atrophy [15] and can confirm the initial diagnosis. The prognosis for vision is poor in all cases. Minimal improvement with anti-inflammatories may occur in the acute phases of the injury but is uncommon.

The ability to assess, initiate treatment, and provide prognoses for various types of ophthalmic emergencies is necessary for the equine emergency clinician. Given the frequency at which orbital injuries or ulcerative keratitis is a reason for equine emergency admissions, it is important to have an appropriate level of familiarity with the management of such cases. It is optimal for such patients to be assessed by a veterinary ophthalmologist, but this may not always be possible in all referral settings.

References

[1] Brooks DE. Orbital trauma, contusion, and periorbital fractures. In: Ophthalmology for the equine practitioner. Jackson (WY): Teton New Media; 2002. p. 37–8.
[2] Millichamp NJ. Ocular trauma. Vet Clin North Am Equine Pract 1992;8(3):521–36.
[3] Irby NL. Ophthalmology. In: Orsini JA, Divers TJ, editors. Manual of equine emergencies. 2nd edition. Philadelphia: Saunders; 2003. p. 436–72.
[4] Irby NL. Nerve blocks of the eye. In: Orsini JA, Divers TJ, editors. Manual of equine emergencies. 2nd edition. Philadelphia: Saunders; 2003. p. 114–6.
[5] Capaldo F, Komáromy AM. Ophthalmic emergency. Current Techniques in Equine Practice 2006;5(2):134–45.
[6] Gum GG, Gelatt KN, Ofri R. Physiology of the eye. In: Gelatt KN, editor. Veterinary ophthalmology. 3rd edition. Philidelphia: Lippincott Williams and Wilkins; 1999. p. 151–83.
[7] Carastro SM. Equine ocular anatomy and ophthalmic examination. Vet Clin North Am Equine Pract 2004;20:285–99.
[8] Van der Woerdt SN. Effects of sedatives on intraocular pressure in the horse. Am J Vet Res 1995;56:155–8.
[9] Caron JP, Barber SM, Bailey JV, et al. Periorbital skull fractures in five horses. J Am Vet Med Assoc 1986;188(3):280–4.
[10] DeBowes RM. Fractures of the cranium. In: Nixon AJ, editor. Equine fracture repair. 1st edition. Philadelphia: W.B. Saunders; 1996. p. 313–22.
[11] Brooks DE. Equine ophthalmology. In: Gelatt KN, editor. Veterinary ophthalmology. 3rd edition. Philadelphia: Lippincott Williams and Wilkins; 1999. p. 1053–116.
[12] Skarda RT. Local anesthetics and local anesthetic techniques in horses. In: Muir WW, Hubbell JAE, editors. Equine anesthesia: monitoring and emergency therapy. St. Louis (MO): Mosby Year Book; 1991. p. 199–246.
[13] Chmielewski NT, Brooks DE, Smith PJ, et al. Visual outcome and ocular survival following iris prolapse in the horse: a review of 32 cases. Equine Vet J 1997;29(1):31–9.

[14] Lavach JD, Severin GA, Roberts SM. Lacerations of the equine eye: a review of 48 cases. J Am Vet Med Assoc 1984;184:1243–8.
[15] Andrews SE, Willis AM. Diseases of the cornea and sclera. In: Gilger BC, editor. Equine ophthalmology. St. Louis (MO): Elsevier Saunders; 2005. p. 157–251.
[16] Brooks DE, Andrew SE, Biros DJ, et al. Ulcerative keratitis caused by beta-hemolytic *Streptococcus equi* in 11 horses. Vet Ophthalmol 2000;3:121–5.
[17] Schoster JV. The assembly and placement of ocular lavage systems in horses. Vet Med 1992; 87:460–71.
[18] Guiliano EA, Maggs DJ, Moore CP, et al. Inferomedial placement of a single-entry subpalpebral lavage tube for treatment of equine eye disease. Vet Ophthalmol 2000;3:153–6.
[19] Sweeney CR, Russell GE. Complications associated with use of a one-hole subpalpebral lavage system in horses: 150 cases (1977–1996). J Am Vet Med Assoc 1997;211:1271–4.
[20] McLaughlin SA, Brightman AH, Helper LC, et al. Pathogenic bacteria and fungi associated with extraocular disease in the horse. J Am Vet Med Assoc 1983;182:241–2.
[21] Sweeney CR, Irby NL. Topical treatment of Pseudomonas sp-infected corneal ulcers in horses: 70 cases (1977–1994). J Am Vet Med Assoc 1996;209:954–7.
[22] Keller RL, Hendrix DVH. Bacterial isolates and antimicrobial susceptibilities in equine bacterial ulcerative keratitis (1993–2004). Equine Vet J 2005;37(3):207–11.
[23] Sauer P, Andrew SE, Lassaline M, et al. Changes in antibiotic resistance in equine bacterial ulcerative keratitis (1991–2000): 65 horses. Vet Ophthalmol 2003;6(4):309–13.
[24] Ollivier FJ, Brooks DE, Van Setten GB, et al. Profiles of matrix metalloproteinase activity in equine tear fluid during corneal healing in 10 horses with ulcerative keratitis. Vet Ophthalmol 2004;7(6):397–405.
[25] Williams MM, Spiess BM, Pascoe PJ, et al. Systemic effects of topical and subconjunctival ophthalmic atropine in the horse. Vet Ophthalmol 2000;3:193–9.
[26] Grahn B, Wolfer J, Keller C, et al. Equine keratomycosis: clinical and laboratory findings in 23 cases. Progress in Veterinary and Comparative Ophthalmology 1993;3:2–7.
[27] Andrew SE, Brooks DE, Smith PJ, et al. Equine ulcerative keratomycosis: visual outcome and ocular survival in 39 cases (1987-1996). Equine Vet J 1998;30:109–16.
[28] Brooks DE, Andrew SE, Dillavou CL. Antimicrobial susceptibility patterns of fungi isolated from horses with ulcerative keratomycosis. Am J Vet Res 1998;59(2):138–42.
[29] Clode AB, Davis JL, Salmon J, et al. Evaluation of concentration of voriconazole in aqueous humor after topical and oral administration in horses. Am J Vet Res 2006;67(2):296–301.
[30] Denis HM. Equine corneal surgery and transplantation. Vet Clin North Am Equine Pract 2004;20:361–80.
[31] Reppas GP, Hodgson DR, McClintock SA, et al. Trauma-induced blindness in two horses. Aust Vet J 1995;72:270–2.

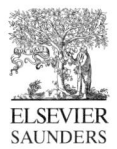

Thoracic Trauma in Horses

Diana M. Hassel, DVM, PhD

Equine Emergency Surgery and Critical Care, Colorado State University, 300 West Drake Road, Fort Collins, CO 80526, USA

Thoracic trauma represents an important cause of morbidity in mortality after injury in human beings and animals. After any form of suspected chest wall trauma, initial emergency management should include assurance of a patent airway and adequate ventilation, along with treatment for shock if present. As with any open wound, tetanus prophylaxis should be instituted. Types of trauma to the thoracic region of the horse include pectoral and axillary lacerations, penetrating chest wounds, flail chest, fractures of the ribs, blunt thoracic trauma, and several potential sequelae that include pneumothorax, pneumomediastinum, hemothorax, pleuritis, fistulae of the sternum or ribs, and diaphragmatic hernia. Emergency management of these various forms of thoracic trauma is discussed.

Pectoral and axillary lacerations

Lacerations to the pectoral and axillary region are common in horses and are often a result of the horse running into various objects, such as fencing or barbed wire; being impaled by sharp objects, such as fence posts or sticks (Figs. 1 and 2); or being kicked by other horses. The large amount of musculature with its extensive blood supply in the region seems to facilitate healing of large wounds and allows a cosmetic outcome, even with extensive wounds.

Wounds of the pectoral and axillary region should be treated as other wounds, beginning with aseptic preparation and exploration of wound depth, with special attention directed at determining involvement of the elbow joint, cranial mediastinum, or cranial thorax. Wound debridement and thorough lavage should follow, but overuse of high-pressure pulsatile lavage should be avoided to prevent dissemination of contaminants into deep fascial planes [1]. Debris deep within the wound should be identified and

E-mail address: dhassel@colostate.edu

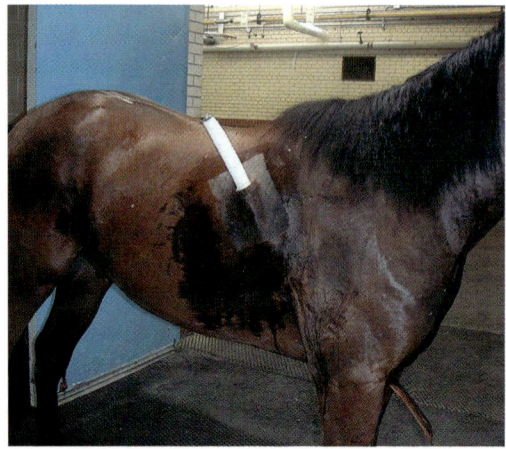

Fig. 1. Penetrating wooden stick enters the right axilla and exits the right hemithorax. (*Courtesy of* Josie Traub-Dargatz, DVM, MS, Fort Collins, CO.)

removed. In most wounds, application of tension sutures, with allowance of adequate drainage in the most ventral aspect, is appropriate. Large avulsive wounds with loss of large amounts of skin may be managed by leaving them left open to heal by second intention.

Unique complications that may be associated with these types of wounds include development of subcutaneous emphysema (Fig. 3), pneumomediastinum, and pneumothorax [2]. Deep wounds in the axilla and pectoral region are particularly prone to these potentially life-threatening complications. Deep penetrating objects, such as fence posts or wooden stakes, may be driven directly into the cranial thorax and mediastinum, resulting in pneumothorax and pneumomediastinum [3]. More commonly,

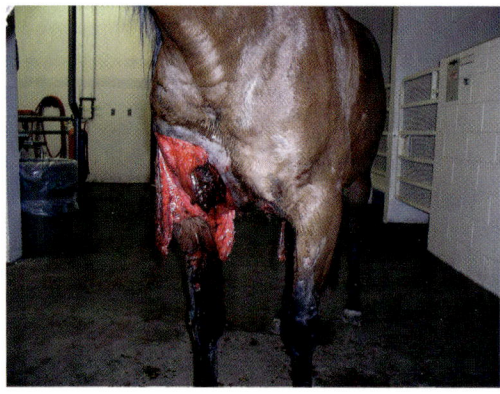

Fig. 2. Right axillary laceration from impact with a fence. (*Courtesy of* Sam Hendrix, DVM, Fort Collins, CO.)

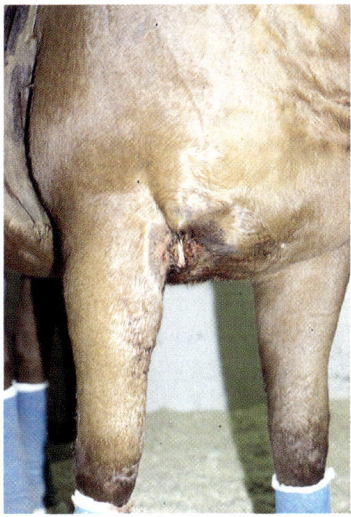

Fig. 3. Subcutaneous emphysema secondary to an axillary wound. (*Courtesy of* Laurie Goodrich, DVM, PhD, Fort Collins, CO.)

axillary wounds may trap air with movement of the forelimbs. To avoid progressive accumulation of air within the soft tissues, limiting movement and temporary occlusion of the wound using stent bandages may be indicated in patients developing subcutaneous emphysema. Trapped subcutaneous air may migrate through fascial planes, with the potential to migrate into the pleural space and mediastinum.

The presence of foreign material in the deepest aspects of the wound often leads to persistent draining tract formation. Diagnostic ultrasound and radiography using contrast fistulography often are necessary to identify the presence of foreign material in chronically infected wound tracts.

Penetrating chest wounds

When presented with a horse with a penetrating wound of the thorax, historical factors of interest should include the mechanism of injury, along with the onset and progression of symptoms. Physical examination should include auscultation and observation of the chest wall for several full respiratory cycles to detect evidence of splinting, paradoxical movement of the chest wall segment, or obvious bony deformities [4]. Palpation may reveal fractures, flail segments, point tenderness, or subcutaneous emphysema. Further evaluation for the detection of nondisplaced fractures, soft tissue injury, hemothorax, and pneumothorax can be performed by means of the use of thoracic ultrasound. Because delays in the development of pneumothorax and hemothorax are commonly encountered, serial evaluations should be performed to identify progressive changes in function [4]. When full-thickness penetration into the pleural cavity is suspected, laboratory assessment should include arterial blood gas determination. This can aid in determining the need for mechanical ventilation in patients with pulmonary contusion or flail chest. Pulse oximetry can also be used as a continuous indicator of the degree of injury and response to treatment [4].

With the presence of a penetrating chest wound, thoracic radiographs may be indicated to identify whether pneumothorax, pneumomediastinum, or concurrent pulmonary or pleural complications exist [4]. Prompt treatment of these serious complications is essential to a successful outcome in these patients. After occlusion of the wound, early placement of a dorsally located chest tube or 10- to 14-gauge intravenous catheter in the 12th intercostal space, with aspiration of pleural air, can provide immediate relief to a horse with a penetrating chest wound with pneumothorax resulting in ventilatory impairment. Use of a three-way stopcock or mechanical suction device may facilitate evacuation of air from the pleural space.

Probing or exploration of chest wall injuries should be exercised with caution. Initial treatment of a contaminated penetrating thoracic wound may consist of limited debridement, gentle lavage, and daily packing of the wound with a sterile hypertonic saline dressing (Curasalt, Kendall Products, Mansfield, Massachusetts) covered by a stent bandage to allow self-debridement and sealing of the wound. If permanent or temporary closure of an open chest wound is possible, this can prevent further aspiration of air into the pleural or other cavities. The application of a plastic material to the outer surface of the wound has been described as a means of providing an airtight seal to reduce influx of air into the pleural cavity [5]. Systemic antibiotics, nonsteroidal anti-inflammatory drugs, and tetanus prophylaxis are also indicated in most cases.

The development of pleuritis or pleuropneumonia is a common sequela to open thoracic wounds [6]; therefore, serial monitoring with appropriate antimicrobial therapy is appropriate. The principles of management of cases of pleuritis secondary to penetrating thoracic wounds are similar to those for acute pleuropneumonia, although bacterial isolates may differ, and inclusion of antimicrobials with a good anaerobic spectrum is important in the management of any infectious disease of the pleural space [6]. If pleural fluid accumulation is identified, intermittent or continuous drainage of the pleural cavity with a closed-suction drain or Heimlich valve may be appropriate (Fig. 4).

Flail chest

Flail chest is rarely observed in the adult horse and is defined as three or more consecutive ribs that are each fractured in at least two sites, resulting in a free-floating segment of the chest wall and paradoxical respiration characterized by inward displacement during inspiration and outward

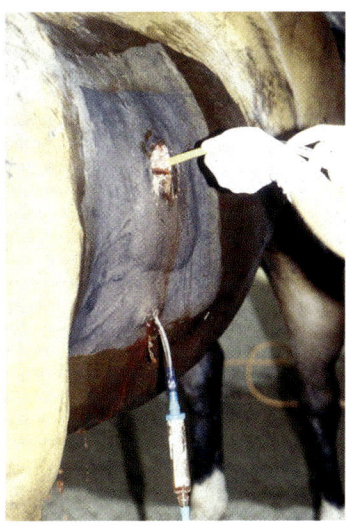

Fig. 4. Thoracic drain with Heimlich valve for treatment of pleuritis secondary to a penetrating thoracic wound. (*Courtesy of* Laurie Goodrich, DVM, PhD, Fort Collins, CO.)

displacement during expiration [7]. Diagnosis is made by physical examination and thorough observation of the respiratory cycle. The defect results in abnormalities of ventilation, oxygenation, and compliance and is typically a consequence of direct impact with a blunt object [4]. Diagnosis of flail chest may be rare in the horse, because the degree of trauma necessary to create flail chest is often rapidly fatal; therefore, a diagnosis may never be made. Severe respiratory dysfunction often occurs as a consequence of flail chest, and increased understanding of the pathophysiology of flail chest has redirected focus from the unstable flail segment to underlying pulmonary damage (eg, contusion) as the primary cause of respiratory dysfunction [8,9]. Described treatment in human patients for flail chest includes aggressive pulmonary physiotherapy, effective analgesia, selective use of endotracheal intubation and ventilation, and close observation for respiratory decompensation [4]. The following criteria may be used as objective guidelines for indication of respiratory failure and the need for endotracheal intubation and mechanical ventilation: clinical signs of progressive respiratory fatigue, tachypnea, or bradypnea; PaO_2 less than 60 mm Hg at an inspired oxygen concentration (FIO_2) greater than 0.5; $PaCO_2$ greater than 55 mm Hg at an FIO_2 greater than 0.5; PaO_2-to-FIO_2 ratio less than 200; clinical evidence of severe shock; associated severe head injury with a need to ventilate; or a severe associated injury requiring surgery [4]. If severe respiratory impairment is not present, attentive observation is indicated, including supplemental oxygen to maintain oxygen saturation at greater than 90% with humidification of inspired air, nutritional support, analgesia, and continuous reassessment. In human beings, surgical stabilization of flail segments is occasionally indicated when a fixed thoracic impaction is present, when there is a failure to wean from mechanical ventilation because of massive chest wall instability, or when the patient is undergoing thoracotomy for treatment of concurrent conditions [4].

Rib fractures

Fractures of the ribs in adult horses may be a component of closed or open chest trauma, such as that attributable to falls, kicks, and road traffic accidents. Comminuted fractures have the potential to injure the lung and pleural cavity, resulting in complications like pneumothorax, hemothorax, and pleuropneumonia [10]. In people, upper rib fractures have been associated with aortic rupture and lower rib fractures with injuries to the spleen and liver [7]. Diagnosis is by means of physical examination, radiography, and ultrasound. Physical examination may reveal a depressed segment of the rib cage or hematoma if the intercostal vasculature was concurrently damaged. Acute rib fractures may appear radiographically as cracks, marginal steps, or obvious discontinuities, whereas chronic fractures are typically identified by callus formation [3]. In adult horses, radiographic identification of rib fractures may be difficult because of the large mass of tissue being penetrated and high milliamperes required to delineate bone from underlying soft tissue structures. Thorough ultrasonographic examination of the surface of each rib is a sensitive method to identify minimally displaced and nondisplaced fractures as well as concurrent soft tissue damage and pleural involvement [11]. Treatment for rib fractures in adult horses consists of management of secondary sequelae, such as hemothorax, pneumothorax, pleuritis, and pulmonary contusions; wound care; and appropriate use of analgesia. Methods for analgesia include the use of opioid analgesics, such as morphine (0.05–0.1 mg/kg administered intravenously every 12–24 hours) [12]; however, morphine should be used with caution at higher doses because of its potential to affect gastrointestinal motility, resulting in colic. Profound analgesia may be obtained when morphine is combined with α_2-agonists, such as xylazine or detomidine [12]. Other systemically administered opioids may include Fentanyl patches (40 µg/kg administered percutaneously every 72 hours) [13,14] or butorphanol as a continuous rate intravenous infusion (13 µg/kg/h) [15] or intermittently administered intravenously or intramuscularly (0.01–0.02 mg/kg every 4–6 hours). Local anesthesia of intercostal nerves with a long-acting anesthetic, such as bupivacaine or mepivacaine, along the caudal surfaces of affected ribs may also provide temporary pain relief.

Rib fractures in foals as a consequence of parturition are a common and potentially fatal event. In a postmortem analysis of 760 newborn foals, 67 had evidence of thoracic trauma; of these, 19 had fractured ribs that were believed to be the cause of death [16]. A separate study evaluating thoracic trauma in foals on a large Thoroughbred breeding farm described 55 foals with thoracic cage asymmetry of 263 examined. These foals were more likely to have a history of abnormal parturition and to have a primiparous dam [17]. The most common sites of injury in foals are the costochondral junction and area immediately above it, with the third to eighth ribs being most frequently affected [16]. Causes of death secondary to rib fracture in foals include hemothorax with subsequent pulmonary collapse, myocardial lacerations or punctures, pulmonary contusion, pneumothorax, diaphragmatic herniation, hemoabdomen, or hemopericardium [16]. Clinical signs that may be observed in foals with rib fractures are highly variable and may include increased lethargy and recumbency, groaning or grunting, plaques of subcutaneous edema overlying the ribs or on the ventral thorax, flinching when the thoracic cage is palpated, and audible or palpable crepitation or clicking when the hand is pressed over the affected region [11].

Foals with existing extensive internal thoracic trauma resulting from rib fractures or the potential for such trauma, which were previously considered to have a guarded to poor prognosis for survival, may be successfully managed with internal fixation of selected fracture sites. Fractured ribs in foals may be successfully reduced and stabilized using reconstruction plates, self-tapping cortical screws, and cerclage wire [18]. Treatment for foals with rib fractures with a reduced risk of life-threatening sequelae (ie, occurring distant from the heart or at costochondral junctions) is early detection and complete stall rest for at least 2 weeks. Local hemorrhage and edema are likely to result in fibrosis and containment of the fractured ends over time. In foals with more severe injuries, analgesia, thoracocentesis, nasal insufflation of oxygen, whole blood transfusions, or sedation and positive-pressure ventilation may be necessary components of treatment.

Rib and sternal fistulae

Fistulae of the rib or sternum may occur as a consequence of osteomyelitis and bone sequestrum formation after open trauma to the region. Diagnosis is straightforward and is determined by means of detection of a fistulous tract and a history of prior trauma to the region. Ultrasonographic and radiographic evaluation with contrast tract injection can provide further insight and may help to differentiate the presence of a foreign body within the deep tissues versus a sequestrum. Treatment consists of surgical exploration and aggressive debridement of the fistulous tract, with subsequent removal of the foreign material or infected tissue. Methods that may facilitate surgical debridement include pre- or intraoperative ultrasonographic guidance to identify the location of the foreign material or sequestrum. Injection of new methylene blue dye into the fistulous tract to demarcate all regions that communicate with the fistula may facilitate complete debridement of infected tissue.

Once removal of the offending foreign body or sequestrum has occurred, healing of rib fistulas is often rapid and successful. Resolution of sternal fistulae carries a guarded prognosis, however, because of the persistence of purulent foci that were undetected at the time of surgery [10].

Pneumothorax

Pneumothorax is a potentially life-threatening injury that can be a complication of any deep injury to the thoracic wall. It has also been associated with other forms of trauma to the respiratory tract, including closed thoracic trauma; as a sequela to pleuropneumonia; as a complication of surgical procedures performed on the respiratory tract; and in association with diaphragmatic hernia [19]. Because the mediastinum of horses is generally described as incomplete, with small fenestrations in the caudal and ventral portions, the development of bilateral pneumothorax might be anticipated with acute open thoracic wounds. Clinical observations suggest that horses with an accumulation of fluid and inflammatory exudate, such as horses with chronic pleuropneumonia, more commonly have unilateral pneumothorax, however [19]. Diagnosis and serial monitoring of pneumothorax may be readily accomplished with thoracic radiography (Fig. 5). On thoracic auscultation, horses with pneumothorax may have absent or dulled breath sounds dorsally, such as may be observed ventrally in horses with pleural effusions.

A tension pneumothorax may form in rare instances. This occurs when a flap of skin or soft tissue acts as a one-way valve, allowing air into the pleural cavity on inspiration but preventing its escape on expiration. This is a rapidly progressive form of pneumothorax that severely compromises respiration and can lead to death [20]. Tension pneumothorax may also develop with a closed pneumothorax as a consequence of a parenchymal

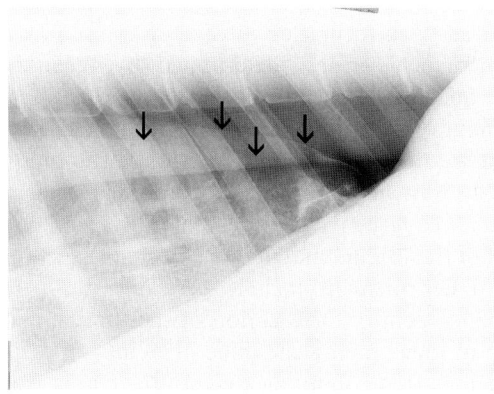

Fig. 5. Lateral thoracic radiograph of a horse with bilateral pneumothorax. Note the complete absence of the pulmonary parenchyma and hyperlucency within the caudodorsal lung fields. Arrows outline the dorsal margins of the right and left lung lobes.

laceration that leaks when the lung undergoes expansion on inspiration [20]. Clinical characteristics of tension pneumothorax may consist of severe respiratory distress, tachycardia, hypotension, and absent breath sounds [7]. Aspiration of air from a dorsally located thoracostomy tube in or near the 12th intercostal space is diagnostic and therapeutic for tension pneumothorax. The thoracic trocar or catheter must be left in place, with periodic aspiration of air until the source of air entry has been sealed.

Chest trochars may be placed using the following method. A site for insertion of the trochar or catheter is selected based on ultrasound guidance if the goal is drainage of accumulated fluid within the pleural cavity or at the dorsal 12th intercostal space for management of pneumothorax. The area is clipped, surgically prepared, and blocked with a local anesthetic. A vertical incision is made in the skin just cranial to the proposed site of entry for placement of larger diameter trochars, such as those used for management of chronic pleuropneumonia. The tip of the trochar is placed through the skin incision and moved to a site between the two ribs and is subsequently inserted into the pleural cavity. Care must be taken to avoid the caudal border of the rib to avoid injury to intercostal vasculature, and guarding of the cannula is essential during placement to avoid overly aggressive insertion into the thorax, resulting in trauma to lung or cardiac tissue. When entry into the pleural cavity has been confirmed by means of aspiration of abnormally accumulated fluid or air, the open end must be aseptically sealed using a Heimlich one-way valve or suction device. The chest tube may be held in place with sutures using a Chinese finger-trap pattern.

Pneumomediastinum

The mediastinum consists of the space between the right and left pleural cavities and is bounded by the mediastinal pleura. Contents of the mediastinum include the trachea, esophagus, heart and great vessels, nerves, lymph nodes, and thoracic duct. Pneumomediastinum has been reported in horses as a consequence of extensive subcutaneous emphysema secondary to an axillary wound [2] and as a consequence of pulmonary bulla formation and subcutaneous emphysema in a neonatal foal [21]. Direct invasion of the mediastinum by means of a penetrating wound of the axilla, caudal neck region, or thorax is an additional potential route of entry for air into the mediastinal space. Alternatively, pneumomediastinum may be observed with conditions like perforation of the thoracic esophagus or tracheal rupture. Classic radiographic features of pneumomediastinum include visualization of the esophagus, great vessels, and outer margins of the trachea (Fig. 6).

There is no specific treatment for pneumomediastinum beyond treatment of the underlying cause, preventing infection with the use of antimicrobial agents, and monitoring closely for the development of pneumothorax.

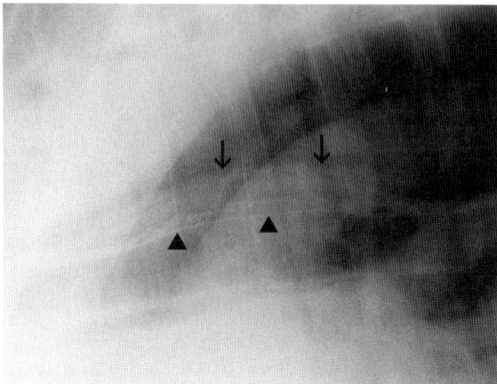

Fig. 6. Lateral thoracic radiograph of a horse with pneumomediastinum. Note the ability to visualize the esophagus (*arrows*) and the outer surface of the trachea (*arrowheads*).

Diaphragmatic hernia

Acquired diaphragmatic hernias may occur as a consequence of trauma to the thorax or abdominal cavity. Blunt trauma to the thorax or abdomen is a common cause of diaphragmatic hernia in people [22]. Other commonly reported causes are situations resulting in an increase in intra-abdominal pressure, such as after a fall, parturition (particularly dystocia), or recent strenuous activity [23]. Horses with diaphragmatic rents can have varied clinical signs, such as exercise intolerance, respiratory compromise, tachypnea [24], or colic secondary to nonstrangulating or strangulating obstruction of a segment of intestine through the diaphragmatic rent [25–27]. Acute abdominal pain is the most common clinical sign, which is related to the severity of displacement of viscera through the rent and subsequent development of obstructions [27]. A lack of palpable abdominal viscera on transrectal palpation may also be identified in some horses with extensive migration of viscera into the thoracic cavity [28]. Often, the diagnosis of diaphragmatic hernia is made at the time of surgery as a result of difficulty with identification of the defect because of its location along the diaphragm or lack of preoperative assessment of the thoracic cavity in a horse with severe signs of colic. Preoperative diagnosis of a diaphragmatic hernia may be facilitated by means of the use of thoracic ultrasonography and thoracic radiography. Thoracic radiographs may reveal the presence of gas-filled intestine or abdominal viscera within the thoracic cavity (Fig. 7), which is pathognomonic for a diaphragmatic hernia. More subtle radiographic abnormalities may be present, such as an inability to visualize the complete cranial margins of the diaphragm or cranial displacement of a portion of the diaphragm. Alternatively, thoracic radiography may not provide any definitive findings supporting a diagnosis of diaphragmatic hernia [29]. Thoracic ultrasonography

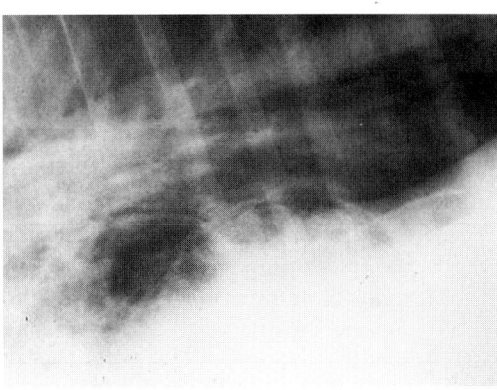

Fig. 7. Lateral thoracic radiograph of a horse with a diaphragmatic hernia with gas-filled large intestine contained within the thoracic cavity.

may provide additional diagnostic clues, depending on the location of the entrapped bowel. An air-filled lung limits sonographic evaluation of the most ventral portion of the diaphragm, but the presence of a pleural effusion may facilitate evaluation as a consequence of dorsal displacement of lung. The curved shape of the diaphragm precludes its complete evaluation, however, even in the presence of pleural fluid [29,30]. Presurgical diagnosis of a diaphragmatic hernia is sometimes difficult, and a definitive diagnosis is most often obtained at the time of surgery or necropsy [29]. In human patients with a diaphragmatic rupture secondary to blunt trauma, similar difficulties in diagnosis have been observed, including lack of identification of the defect during surgical exploration [22]. Laparoscopy or thoracoscopy can also be used to diagnose diaphragmatic hernias. It is important to have suction available to reinflate the thorax, however, if a diaphragmatic hernia is present and the horse shows any sign of distress [31].

Successful surgical repair of diaphragmatic hernias has been reported in adult horses and foals [23,32–35], and horses can successfully return to high levels of performance and deliver foals after repair [32]. Repair of diaphragmatic defects is often a surgical challenge, however, because the defects are often inaccessible from a standard ventral midline celiotomy approach to the abdomen. Described methods for repair include direct repair by means of suturing [32] or mesh application from a ventral midline celiotomy if the defect is surgically accessible by means of extension of the ventral midline incision or thoracotomy [27,31] and delayed repair using a lateral approach to the thorax with thoracic rib resection and thoracoscopy [28,36]. Reported complications include breakdown of the site of hernia repair during recovery from anesthesia [26]; rupture of the diaphragm ventral to the original rent at a later date [37]; and anesthetic complications, including pronounced hypoxemia, hypercapnia [32], and ineffective positive-pressure ventilation [38].

Blunt chest trauma

Blunt forces applied to the chest wall cause injury by three mechanisms: rapid deceleration (eg, motor vehicle injuries in people), direct impact, and compression [4]. The most common injuries in human beings after blunt chest trauma are thoracic cage fractures, lung contusions and tears, myocardial contusions, and aortic rupture [7]. Massive pulmonary embolism characterized by late-onset progressive dyspnea [39] and tracheal injuries [40] have also been reported. These complications are rarely observed in the adult horse, however. Fractures of the ribs with or without associated hemothorax and pulmonary contusions are likely to be a sequela of blunt trauma in the adult horse secondary to direct impact, such as that from a motor vehicle, a kick from another horse, or running into a stationary object. Flail chest is another rare but potential sequela to extensive blunt thoracic trauma. In foals, blunt trauma may occur as a consequence of dystocia or perhaps as a result of thoracic compression from being stepped on by an adult horse. Treatment for blunt thoracic trauma depends on the associated injuries and presence or absence of respiratory compromise.

Summary

Management of horses with a history of trauma to the thoracic region should begin with physical examination, noting the attitude of the horse, character of respiration, and manner of movement. If respiratory distress is present, emergency management to determine and resolve the source of distress is indicated. Early assessment of the pleural cavity with the use of ultrasound or radiography to identify the presence or absence of pleural fluid or gas accumulation allows prompt treatment and resolution of a life-threatening respiratory impairment. In the absence of these diagnostic modalities, thorough auscultation and percussion of the thorax may reveal the presence or absence of pleural fluid or pneumothorax. Management of shock with appropriate volume resuscitation is also appropriate on initial presentation. With penetrating chest wounds, rapid treatment, including dorsal aspiration of free pleural air with a catheter and temporary occlusion of a sucking chest wound, may allow adequate time for transfer to a facility prepared to provide serial monitoring of respiratory function. This may include ongoing arterial blood gas assessment and surgical management of large open thoracic wounds with provision of positive-pressure ventilation. Once stable, a more thorough assessment of the horse is appropriate to identify the presence of concurrent injuries, such as rib fractures, diaphragmatic hernia, hemothorax, pleuritis, and the presence of foreign material within the wound. Axillary wounds should be evaluated for their potential to trap air, resulting in subcutaneous emphysema with the potential for the development of pneumomediastinum and pneumothorax.

References

[1] Stashak TS. Wounds of the body. In: Stashak TS, editor. Equine wound management. Malvern (PA): Lea & Febiger; 1991. p. 278.
[2] Hance SR, Robertson JT. Subcutaneous emphysema from an axillary wound that resulted in pneumomediastinum and bilateral pneumothorax in a horse. J Am Vet Med Assoc 1992; 200(8):1107–10.
[3] Farrow CS. Veterinary diagnostic imaging: the horse. St. Louis (MO): Elsevier Mosby; 2006.
[4] Moore EE, Feliciano DV, Mattox KL. Trauma manual. 4th edition. New York: McGraw-Hill Medical Pub. Division; 2003.
[5] Reed SM, Bayly WM, Sellon DC. Equine internal medicine. 2nd edition. Philadelphia: W.B. Saunders; 2004.
[6] Collins MB, Hodgson DR, Hutchins DR. Pleural effusion associated with acute and chronic pleuropneumonia and pleuritis secondary to thoracic wounds in horses: 43 cases (1982–1992). J Am Vet Med Assoc. 1994;205(12):1753–8.
[7] Naudé GP, Demetriades D. Trauma secrets. 2nd edition. Philadelphia: Elsevier Health Sciences; 2003.
[8] Olsen D, Renberg W, Perrett J, et al. Clinical management of flail chest in dogs and cats: a retrospective study of 24 cases (1989–1999). J Am Anim Hosp Assoc 2002;38(4):315–20.
[9] Bjorling D. Surgical management of flail chest. In: Bojrab MJ, Ellison GW, Slocum B, editors. Current techniques in small animal surgery. 4th edition. Baltimore (MD): Williams & Wilkins; 1998. p. 421–4.
[10] Wintzer H-J. Equine diseases: a textbook for students and practitioners. Berlin (NY): P Parey; Springer-Verlag; 1986.
[11] Sprayberry KA, Bain FT, Seahorn TL, et al. Fifty-six cases of rib fractures in neonatal foals hospitalized in a referral center intensive care unit from 1997–2001. Presented at the Annual Convention of the American Association of Equine Practitioners. San Diego (CA), November 25–28, 2001.
[12] Muir W. Recognizing and treating pain in horses. In: Reed SM, Bayly WM, Sellon DC, editors. Equine internal medicine. 2nd edition. St. Louis (MO): Elsevier; 2004. p. 1529–41.
[13] Maxwell LK, Thomasy SM, Slovis N, et al. Pharmacokinetics of fentanyl following intravenous and transdermal administration in horses. Equine Vet J 2003;35(5):484–90.
[14] Thomasy SM, Slovis N, Maxwell LK, et al. Transdermal fentanyl combined with nonsteroidal anti-inflammatory drugs for analgesia in horses. J Vet Intern Med 2004;18(4):550–4.
[15] Sellon DC, Roberts MC, Blikslager AT, et al. Effects of continuous rate intravenous infusion of butorphanol on physiologic and outcome variables in horses after celiotomy. J Vet Intern Med 2004;18(4):555–63.
[16] Schambourg MA, Laverty S, Mullim S, et al. Thoracic trauma in foals: post mortem findings. Equine Vet J 2003;35(1):78–81.
[17] Jean D, Laverty S, Halley J, et al. Thoracic trauma in newborn foals. Equine Vet J 1999; 31(2):149–52.
[18] Bellezzo F, Hunt RJ, Provost R, et al. Surgical repair of rib fractures in 14 neonatal foals: case selection, surgical technique and results. Equine Vet J 2004;36(7):557–62.
[19] Boy MG, Sweeney CR. Pneumothorax in horses: 40 cases (1980-1997). J Am Vet Med Assoc 2000;216(12):1955–9.
[20] Kramek BA, Caywood DD. Pneumothorax. Vet Clin North Am Small Anim Pract 1987; 17(2):285–300.
[21] Marble SL, Edens LM, Shiroma JT, et al. Subcutaneous emphysema in a neonatal foal. J Am Vet Med Assoc 1996;208(1):97–9.
[22] Esme H, Solak O, Sahin DA, et al. Blunt and penetrating traumatic ruptures of the diaphragm. Thorac Cardiovasc Surg 2006;54(5):324–7.
[23] Bristol D. Diaphragmatic hernias in horses and cattle. Compendium on Continuing Education for the Practicing Veterinarian 1986;8:S407–11.

[24] Goehring LS, Goodrich LR, Murray MJ. Tachypnoea associated with a diaphragmatic tear in a horse. Equine Vet J 1999;31(5):443–5.
[25] Everett KA, Chaffin MK, Brinsko SP. Diaphragmatic herniation as a cause of lethargy and exercise intolerance in a mare. Cornell Vet 1992;82(3):217–23.
[26] Perdrizet JA, Dill SG, Hackett RP. Diaphragmatic hernia as a cause of dyspnoea in a draft horse. Equine Vet J 1989;21(4):302–4.
[27] Dabareiner RM, White NA. Surgical repair of a diaphragmatic hernia in a racehorse. J Am Vet Med Assoc 1999;214(10):1517–8, 1496.
[28] Malone ED, Farnsworth K, Lennox T, et al. Thoracoscopic-assisted diaphragmatic hernia repair using a thoracic rib resection. Vet Surg 2001;30(2):175–8.
[29] Bryant JE, Sanchez LC, Rameriz S, et al. What is your diagnosis? Herniation of the intestines into the caudal region of the thorax. J Am Vet Med Assoc 2002;220(10):1461–2.
[30] Williams J, Leveille R, Myer C. Imaging modalities used to confirm diaphragmatic hernias in small animals. Compend Cont Educ Pract Vet 1998;20:1199–209.
[31] Fischer AT. Diaphragmatic hernias in the horse. Presented at the American College of Veterinary Surgeons Symposium. San Diego (CA), October 27–29, 2005.
[32] Santschi EM, Juzwiak JS, Moll HD, et al. Diaphragmatic hernia repair in three young horses. Vet Surg 1997;26(3):242–5.
[33] Coffman JR, Kintner LD. Strangulated diaphragmatic hernia in a horse. Vet Med Small Anim Clin 1972;67(4):423–6.
[34] Speirs VC, Reynolds WT. Successful repair of a diaphragmatic hernia in a foal. Equine Vet J 1976;8(4):170–2.
[35] Proudman CJ, Edwards GB. Diaphragmatic diverticulum (hernia) in a horse. Equine Vet J 1992;24(3):244–6.
[36] Vachon AM, Fischer AT. Thoracoscopy in the horse: diagnostic and therapeutic indications in 28 cases. Equine Vet J 1998;30(6):467–75.
[37] Hill FW, Knottenbelt DC, van Laeren K. Repair of a diaphragmatic hernia in a horse. Vet Rec 1987;120(6):127–9.
[38] Branson KR, Kramer J. Anesthesia case of the month. Diaphragmatic hernia making it difficult to ventilate a horse during anesthesia. J Am Vet Med Assoc 2000;216(12):1918–9.
[39] Politi A, Galli M, Ferrari G. [Massive pulmonary embolism after blunt chest trauma: considerations on pathogenesis and therapy]. G Ital Cardiol 1998;28(5):567–70.
[40] Ahmad U, Javed MA, Fatimi SH. Tracheal injury due to blunt chest trauma: a rare surgical emergency. J Coll Physicians Surg Pak 2006;16(6):422–3.

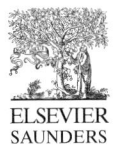

Trauma with Neurologic Sequelae

Brett S. Tennent-Brown, BVSc

Department of Clinical Studies, University of Pennsylvania School of Veterinary Medicine, New Bolton Center, 382 West Street Road, Kennett Square, PA 19348, USA

Injury to the equine spinal column occurs most commonly to the cervical and thoracolumbar vertebrae [1–3]. Causes of spinal trauma in horses include rearing and falling over backward, collisions with solid objects or other animals, kicks, and slipping on unsure footing. Fractures of the cervical spine are most commonly reported in immature horses and may occur during halter training or while playing (Figs. 1–3). Adult horses may injure the cervical or thoracolumbar region in high-speed paddock accidents or during athletic events, particularly those involving jumping. Thoracolumbar fractures are observed more commonly in adult horses than in foals. Fracture of the sacrum and caudal (coccygeal) vertebrae can occur when a horse sits violently backward on the ground or against a solid object.

The pathogenesis and clinical signs associated with brain injury after head trauma and peripheral nerve injury have been excellently described recently [4,5]. Management of the recumbent horse has also been well described [6,7]. This review therefore concentrates on the pathologic findings and clinical signs associated with acute spinal cord injury (SCI) and the initial treatment of those patients.

Pathophysiology

The pathophysiology of SCI comprises primary and secondary injuries [8]. Primary injury occurs as a result of mechanical forces imparted to the cord and consists of severed axons, physical damage to neurons and glial cells, and disruption of the microvasculature. Secondary injury refers to the cascade of events that follow the primary insult, including microvascular ischemia, oxidative stress, excitotoxicity, ion dysregulation, and inflammation [8]. These secondary processes act synergistically to disturb neuroglial architecture further through cell death and extend injury beyond the initial

---

E-mail address: tennentb@vet.upenn.edu

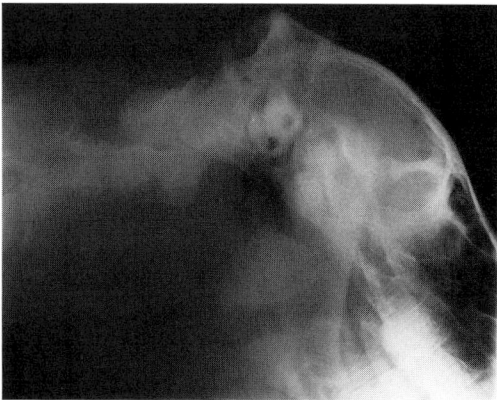

Fig. 1. Lateral radiograph of the cervical spine of a 5-month-old colt presented for trauma. There is dorsal and cranial subluxation of the dens, with narrowing of the spinal canal dorsal to the dens.

epicenter. It is often the severity of secondary injury that limits the restoration of neurologic function and determines the prognosis [9].

In human beings, SCI may be initiated by one of the following insults to the neuroparenchyma: impact with transient or permanent compression, distraction and forcible stretching of the spinal cord or its blood supply, and laceration and transaction [9]. Injury to the equine spinal cord most commonly occurs as the osteoligamentous spinal column fails subsequent

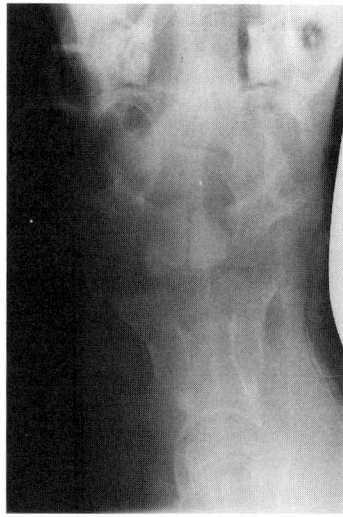

Fig. 2. Ventrodorsal radiograph of the cervical spine in the same horse as in Fig. 1. There is malalignment of the vertebral bodies that appears to be centered on the right side of the dens at the level of the physis, consistent with a Salter-Harris fracture.

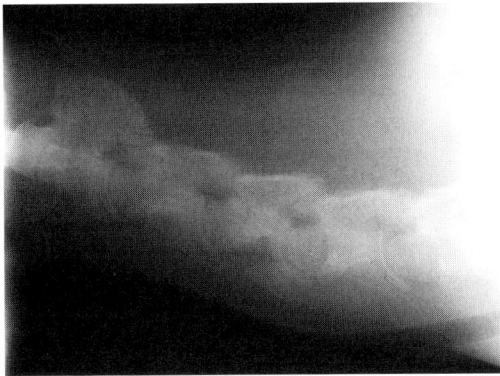

Fig. 3. Lateral radiograph of the cervical spine of a 2.5-month-old filly presented for trauma. There is a comminuted fracture of the fourth cervical vertebra involving the body and caudal epiphysis as well as the spinal canal. Spinal cord compression and hemorrhage were evident on the subsequent postmortem examination. Ventral deviation of the trachea in the region of the fourth and fifth vertebrae represents soft tissue swelling ventral to the fracture site.

to falls or collisions, and compression of the cord is probably most common [1]. Penetrating wounds and laceration of the cord occur infrequently in equine practice. The initial mechanical insult tends to damage the central gray matter primarily, with relative sparing of the white matter [10]. The greater propensity of the gray matter to injury during the primary insult may be related to its softer consistency and greater vascularity.

Studies predominantly conducted in animals have helped to elucidate the raft of interrelated processes thought to contribute to secondary SCI. Identifying and understanding these processes is important because they may provide therapeutic targets.

Vascular abnormalities

Alterations in vascular tone and integrity and subsequent ischemia seem to be crucial elements in secondary SCI, although the exact mechanisms by which they occur are unknown. The capillaries and venules of the microcirculation seem to be particularly susceptible and may be damaged cranial and caudal to the site of primary injury [11]. A combination of mechanical disruption, intraparenchymal hemorrhage and edema, thrombosis, and vasospasm leads to profound spinal cord hypoperfusion [12]. Perfusion is usually more severely affected in the gray matter, and the metabolic requirements of the neuron cell bodies make this area extremely sensitive to ischemia [12]. Irreversible damage to the gray matter may occur within the first hour of injury, whereas the white matter seems to be more resistant [13].

Autoregulatory mechanisms normally maintain tight control of the microvasculature within the spinal cord and brain, providing constant perfusion over a range of systemic blood pressures. These mechanisms may be impaired after SCI [14], however, and the spinal cord becomes vulnerable to decreases in systemic blood pressure [15]. Patients with trauma may be hypotensive for several reasons, including hypovolemia secondary to hemorrhage or neurogenic shock. Neurogenic shock, defined as inadequate tissue perfusion secondary to loss of vasomotor input, is characterized by bradycardia and hypotension with decreased peripheral resistance and depressed cardiac output [8]. These effects have been associated with decreased sympathetic tone, increased vagal tone, and changes to the myocardium itself [16].

After a period of hypoperfusion, the cord may undergo reperfusion and hyperemia, which, ironically, can cause more damage than the initial ischemia. Hyperperfusion is thought to result from the perivascular accumulation of waste metabolites and leads to the generation of oxygen-free radicals and other toxic byproducts that further contribute to secondary injury [17].

Free radicals and lipid peroxidation

Free radicals liberated by inflammatory cells and generated during hypoperfusion and reperfusion initiate several damaging reactions [18]. Oxygen-derived free radicals include superoxide, hydroxyl, nitric oxide, and peroxynitrite radicals that may be generated by multiple pathways. When oxidative stress exceeds the endogenous antioxidant capacity, oxidation of proteins, lipids, and nucleic acids ensues. Lipid peroxidation is particularly damaging and initiates a cycle that generates more free radicals and alters the characteristics of the cell membrane. The increased oxidative stress may also disable mitochondrial enzymes, alter DNA and DNA-associated proteins, inactivate membrane sodium channels, and inhibit the Na^+/K^+-ATPase [18]. These pathologic processes combine to induce metabolic collapse and cell death [19].

Excitotoxicity

Subsequent to acute SCI, excitatory neurotransmitters that may cause direct and indirect damage to the cord are released [20,21]. Glutamate is the most abundant excitatory neurotransmitter in the central nervous system (CNS) and is released excessively after cord injury [22]. Indirect damage is thought to result from the production of reactive species and alteration of microvascular function [23].

Direct damage results from the action of excitatory neurotransmitters at ion channels. Glutamate acts at several receptors involved in ion transport and cellular metabolism, including the N-methyl-D-aspartate (NMDA) receptors and α-amino-3-hydroxy-5-methylisoxazolepropionate (AMPA) and kainate receptors [22]. These membrane proteins are, in part, responsible for sodium and calcium ion regulation. Other glutamate receptors participate in a range of cellular functions. Excitotoxicity is defined as the deleterious effects of excess glutamate stimulation at these receptors [21].

Glutamate activation of NMDA receptors allows extracellular calcium (and sodium) ions to move into the cell. Stimulation of the NMDA receptors may also allow the release of calcium ions from cytoplasmic stores [24].

Ion homeostasis dysregulation

Increases in cytosolic and mitochondrial calcium ion concentration are thought to trigger a multitude of processes that lethally alter cellular metabolism [25,26]. These include activation of proteases and lipases, generation of free radicals, and dysregulation of mitochondrial oxidative phosphorylation [9]. Calcium-dependent proteases and kinases destroy specific components of the cell membrane and ultrastructure and attack structural components of the CNS. Interference with mitochondrial function inhibits cellular respiration in a cell already compromised by hypoxia and ischemia. Intracellular calcium accumulation may represent the final common pathway for toxic cell death.

Intracellular sodium influx may result from activation of the NMDA and AMPA and kainate receptors by glutamate. Sodium influx may also occur as a result of activation of voltage-gated sodium channels or activation of a sodium-calcium ion exchanger [9]. Injured neurons lose the ability to pump the sodium ions out of the intracellular compartment; as a consequence, toxic accumulation of sodium and water occurs [27]. Increased extracellular concentrations of potassium may also occur in SCI and seem to result in excessive depolarization of neurons, adversely affecting neuronal conduction. This may be a critical factor underlying spinal shock [28].

Inflammatory and immunologic response

Acutely after SCI, blood-borne neutrophils infiltrate the injury site, releasing a range of substances, including proteolytic enzymes and oxygen free radicals, which may further damage the local tissues [29]. In addition, they secrete an array of cytokines that recruit additional inflammatory cells. As the injury becomes chronic, blood-borne macrophages and resident microglial cells are recruited, both of which phagocytose and remove the damaged tissues [30]. These cells release yet more cytokines, further modulating the immune response [31,32].

Cytokines released by inflammatory cells after spinal cord trauma induce the expression of lipases, lipoxygenases, and cyclooxygenases [33,34]. The lipoxygenases and cyclooxygenases, particularly cyclooxygenase-2 (COX-2), promote the metabolism of arachidonic acid and the elaboration of proinflammatory prostanoids, including prostacyclines, thromboxanes, prostaglandins, and leukotrienes. Excessive cytoplasmic calcium may activate specific phospholipases, augmenting arachidonic acid metabolism. Increased concentrations of excitatory neurotransmitters may also induce COX-2 expression [35].

Matrix metalloproteinases (MMPs) are zinc-dependent endopeptidases with physiologic and pathologic roles and are involved in cord injury and repair. Expression of MMP-9 in a rodent model of SCI is associated with changes in vascular permeability and neutrophil migration [36]. Inhibition of MMPs has been shown to reduce the disruption in the blood–spinal cord barrier and to improve locomotor outcome [36,37]. It was recently demonstrated that MMP-9 expression increased acutely in dogs with intervertebral disk disease and severe neurologic dysfunction [38].

Necrosis and apoptosis

Necrotic and apoptotic cell death has been documented after SCI [39]. Both processes may be activated by the same events: inflammation, ischemia, free radical damage, and excitotoxicity. In general, the more severe the insult, the more likely the cell is to undergo necrosis. In addition, the inflammatory reaction associated with necrosis is generally absent in apoptosis. Cells spared severe trauma during initial injury may accumulate sufficient insults to initiate apoptosis that may occur weeks after and at sites remote to the inciting insult [40,41]. The distinction between necrosis and apoptosis is important because the latter may be amenable to therapeutic intervention [9].

There are two main pathways of apoptosis [8]. Extrinsic (receptor dependent) apoptosis is evoked by extracellular signals, including tumor necrosis factor (TNF), which accumulates rapidly after SCI, and inducible nitric oxide synthase (iNOS). Intrinsic (receptor independent) apoptosis is activated by intracellular signals, including high intracellular calcium concentrations. The extrinsic and intrinsic pathways initiate sequential activation of distinct populations of caspases, which facilitate programmed cell death [42].

Numerous other factors are likely to play a role in secondary neuronal injury and death. Depletion of intracellular magnesium, for example, has been purported to have numerous deleterious effects on cellular metabolism [8]. Mitochondria have been suggested to represent an integral mediator of cellular death after neural injury, and several injury mechanisms involve the mitochondria in some capacity [43]. Finally, the loss or impairment of body function after SCI is mostly permanent, because injured neurons within the CNS have a limited ability to regenerate and regain functional connections. This reflects an intrinsic cellular incompetence and the nonpermissive environment for neuronal growth within the adult mammalian CNS [44,45].

Diagnosis and clinical signs

In an emergency situation, the initial physical examination may be abbreviated and should rapidly aim to determine the preeminent problem and assess the cardiovascular status of the patient [46]. Given the importance of CNS hypoperfusion in the pathogenesis of secondary SCI, assessment of the volume status should be a priority.

A detailed neurologic examination is required to localize the lesion to direct additional diagnostics and formulate a treatment plan [46,47]. To facilitate neuroanatomic localization, the spinal cord has been divided into five regions: (1) high cervical (C1–C5), (2) cervicothoracic (C6–T2), (3) thoracolumbar (T3–L2), (4) lumbosacral (L3–S2), and (5) sacrococcygeal (S3–Cd5) [48]. Animals with spinal cord disease without central involvement usually have an intact sensorium and retain their appetite.

Clinical signs depend on the location of the lesion and the relative amount of damage to the gray (cell bodies) and white (myelinated spinal cord tracts) matter [48]. The white matter is usually more susceptible to compression than the gray matter. Because of the less compressible nature of the gray matter and the high metabolic requirements of the neurons, however, the gray matter is more susceptible to the effects of secondary injury. In general terms, damage to the white matter and disruption of pathways from the brain initiating and controlling voluntary motor function cause clinical signs of upper motor neuron (UMN) disease. Damage to the gray matter results in lower motor neuron (LMN) deficits.

In addition to injury to the cell bodies within the gray matter, LMN signs may occur as a result of damage to any of the structures within the motor portion of the reflex arc. LMN lesions cause signs of muscle weakness (paresis or paralysis), hyporeflexia or areflexia, hypotonia or atonia, and neurogenic atrophy. Spinal reflexes (triceps, biceps, and patella) are depressed or absent with an LMN lesion. Clinical signs of UMN disease include paresis or paralysis, depending on severity. The muscles are usually hypertonic, although hypotonia is occasionally seen, and the spinal reflexes are intact (normal) or hyperactive (hyperreflexia). Sensory losses with an UMN lesion may be proprioceptive or cutaneous. Animals with an UMN lesion may show a withdrawal reflex but no central awareness in response to stimuli applied to the limbs.

Urinary incontinence may result from disruption to the UMN or LMN input to the bladder [49]. SCI above the sacral segments leads to UMN bladder dysfunction, characterized by a turgid bladder and excessive tone of the striated urethral musculature. Attempts to urinate produce small squirts of urine only when intravesicular pressure extends that of the urethral sphincter. Per rectum expression of the bladder is difficult or impossible. Injury affecting the gray matter of the sacral segments results in an LMN bladder characterized by loss of detrusor function (atonia) and urethral relaxation. Urine dribbling is nearly constant, and the bladder is easily expressed during rectal palpation. It should be noted that the distinction between UMN and LMN bladders is not always absolute. Further, loss of detrusor function occurs commonly as a result of chronic dysfunction, and horses with a lesion cranial to the sacral segments may have a bladder more characteristic of an LMN injury [50]. Fecal incontinence results from lesions in the autonomic segments of the sacral spinal cord, causing fecal impaction in the distal rectum.

Cutaneous sensation and the panniculus reflex can be valuable in localizing a focal spinal cord lesion [47,48]. Examination is performed by gently pricking the neck, trunk, and limbs and should be conducted in a caudal-to-cranial direction. Irritation of the skin over the trunk is detected by segmental sensory nerves; the nervous impulse enters the corresponding spinal cord segment and is passed cranially to the T1 and C8 segments. Here, the impulse stimulates the LMN cell bodies of the lateral thoracic nerve, which innervates the cutaneous trunci, causing contraction ("panniculus reflex"). A lesion anywhere along this pathway may interfere with the reflex. Dermatomes immediately caudal to an affected spinal cord segment have decreased cutaneous sensation, and there may be areas of focal sweating. An area of hyperesthesia is occasionally observed in patients with a focal spinal cord segment or nerve root injury. Stoic horses or those with a severe central lesion may not respond as expected to cutaneous stimulation.

High cervical (C1–C5)

Animals with incomplete lesions within this region of the spinal cord display hemiparesis or tetraparesis. Clinical signs may include knuckling, stumbling, and limb interference; crossing over midline and pivoting on the inside foot when turned; hypermetria; abnormal postural placement responses; and excessive truncal sway. Animals with severe high cervical lesions become recumbent and are unable to lift their head from the ground. The righting response is asymmetric in animals with unilateral lesions; these animals can only raise the head and neck when lying with the lesion on the down side. In recumbent animals, muscle tone of the limbs and spinal reflexes are consistent with an UMN lesion. Conscious perception of painful stimuli may be depressed or absent in all limbs. Urination is difficult because of increased urethral sphincter tone (ie, an UMN bladder). Animals with complete spinal cord transection cranial to C6 may die suddenly subsequent to respiratory paralysis.

Cervicothoracic (C6–T2)

Lesions within the brachial intumescence result in tetraparesis or tetraplegia and conscious proprioceptive deficits in all four limbs. The forelimbs are hypotonic and hyporeflexive, consistent with LMN dysfunction. The hind limbs, in contrast, are hypertonic and hyperreflexive as would be expected of an UMN lesion. Unilateral lesions result in ipsilateral signs. Lesions within the C6-to-T2 region may not produce forelimb hypotonia if only the white matter is involved and the gray matter is spared. Conscious perception of painful stimuli may be depressed or absent in all limbs. The righting responses of the head and neck are normal, but these animals are unlikely to be able to achieve sternal recumbency. The bladder is characteristic of UMN disruption, as for high cervical lesions. More chronic lesions affecting the gray matter or nerve roots result in neurogenic atrophy of the associated forelimb muscle groups. Differentiation of high (C1–C5) and low (C6–T2) cervical spinal cord lesions may be difficult in horses, especially when signs are mild.

Gray matter lesions of T1-to-T3 spinal segments may result in Horner's syndrome and loss of sympathetic innervation to the head. In horses, this is characterized by miosis, enophthalmos, nictitans prolapse, and ptosis. Enophthalmos, nictitans prolapse, and ptosis are a result of loss of tone in the periorbital structures. Sweating on the affected side and edema of the nasal mucosa may be apparent.

Thoracolumbar (T3–L2)

Incomplete lesions of the thoracolumbar region (T3–L2 or T3–L3) result in normal activity of the forelimbs and proprioceptive deficits in the hind limbs. Paraplegia occurs with complete lesions in this region, although the animal may be able to assume a "dog-sitting" position. Muscle tone and spinal reflexes of the hind limbs are exaggerated. The urinary bladder has characteristics of UMN dysfunction.

Animals with severe spinal cord insults between T2 and L2 may display transient hypertonia of the forelimbs (Schiff-Sherrington syndrome). This phenomenon is caused by injury to inhibitory fibers that ascend from the lumbar segments and synapse on the forelimb LMN within the brachial intumescence. Forelimb hypertonia as a result of the Schiff-Sherrington syndrome should be accompanied by intact conscious proprioceptive responses in contrast to the hypertonia subsequent to high cervical lesions.

Lumbosacral (L3–S2)

Lesions within the lumbosacral region result in paraparesis or paraplegia of the pelvic limbs. Animals with incomplete lesions show hind limb ataxia and conscious proprioceptive deficits. Patients with complete lesions between L3 and S2 have flaccid paraplegia accompanied by hyporeflexia or areflexia. With prolonged denervation, neurogenic atrophy of the hind limb musculature occurs.

Lesions located between spinal cord segments L3 and L6 result in a urinary bladder characteristics of an UMN lesion. Lesions located around the S1 and S2 segments result in bladder distention and flaccidity with reduced sphincter tone characteristic of LMN injury, however.

Sacrococcygeal (S3–Cd5)

Lesions of the sacrococcygeal region (cauda equina) produce flaccidity of the tail and anus and paraphimosis in male horses. Additionally, there is desensitization of the tail, perineum, anus, and penis or vulva. The urethral sphincter is dilated, and urine constantly drips from the urethral orifice. The animal is unable to urinate or defecate, resulting in a large dilated urinary bladder and distention of the rectum with feces. If the entire neurologic lesion is located caudal to S3, ataxia or conscious proprioceptive deficits are not present.

Cerebrospinal fluid analysis

Cerebrospinal fluid (CSF) analysis is unlikely to provide additional information in a case of spinal trauma but may help to rule out other diagnoses when the cause of neurologic signs is unknown. Samples may be collected from the atlanto-occipital (AO) or lumbosacral space. A general anesthetic is obviously required to acquire an AO sample, and not all horses tolerate a lumbosacral puncture. Therefore, the potential risks and benefits should be carefully considered.

Neuroimaging

The radiographic characteristics of the equine vertebral column have been well described [51]. One should be familiar with the age at which growth plates close and other radiographic features of the equine vertebral column to avoid misinterpretation. It should be recognized that severe SCI can occur without evidence of bony injury. Furthermore, significant SCI may occur a considerable distance from the site of the primary osseous injury as a result of shear forces and soft tissue inflammation. When possible, therefore, it may be worth considering radiographing the entire spinal column, because lesions may be missed with radiographic surveys based on neuroanatomic localization of the lesion alone.

Myelography is a relatively safe, although not completely benign, procedure that can allow more accurate identification of lesions compressing the spinal cord. Although largely restricted to assessment of the cervical spine, the technique has been used to assess the integrity of more caudal structures [2].

The advantages of CT and MRI and their application to equine patients have been described [52]. The major limitation to these procedures is their availability and requirement for a general anesthetic. Currently, there are also physical limitations on what may be practically imaged. In the human field, CT has been shown to be considerably more sensitive for the detection of fractures when compared with plain film radiography [53]. MRI provides the best evaluation of soft tissue pathologic change and is able to evaluate the spinal cord directly. MRI may be used to detect vascular anomalies and to evaluate posttraumatic sequelae. Despite these distinctions, the processes should be regarded as complementary and, in human patients, are often used in combination with plain radiography for complete evaluation of the spinal column [53].

Acute management of the patient with trauma

In human medicine, much of the improvement in outcome from SCI is a consequence of prehospital care [54]. The assumption that all patients with trauma have SCI has led to routine rigid immobilization until the integrity of the spine has been established. Similar immobilization in equine patients is impractical and probably unnecessary because of the extensive muscular splinting of the spinal column in conscious animals. Nevertheless, it would seem prudent to take precautions when possible, particularly in patients with suspected neck injuries and foals with spinal trauma. Recumbent patients may be placed on sheets of plywood or sturdy rubber floor mats with ropes attached at the corners for movement [6]. Heavy-duty plastic sleds are commercially available [55].

Sedation or short-term anesthesia is often required in the initial management of patients with trauma or to perform diagnostic procedures. Acepromazine and ketamine should probably be avoided in animals suspected of having head trauma or at risk for seizures. In healthy conscious horses, the commonly used α_2-adrenergic agonists decrease CSF pressure [56]. Although the effects of these drugs may differ in neurologic disease, they seem to be rational choices for these patients. Xylazine (0.2–1.1 mg/kg administered intravenously) or detomidine (0.005–0.02 mg/kg administered intravenously), alone or in combination with the opioid agonist-antagonist butorphanol (0.044–0.066 mg/kg administered intravenously), provides excellent sedation. The direct effects of opioids on cerebral blood flow (CBF) and intracranial pressure (ICP) are minimal, although they may indirectly increase CSF pressure as a result of respiratory depression and carbon dioxide retention.

Most of the injectable anesthetics, with the exception of the dissociative agents, reduce cerebral metabolic rate of oxygen ($CMRO_2$) requirements, CBF, and ICP [57]. Although the claim that barbiturates may be beneficial in brain injury is widely disputed, they seem unlikely to be of harm aside from prolonging anesthetic recovery. In contrast, volatile anesthetics increase CBF and alter the $CMRO_2$ to varying degrees [57]. Respiratory depression and carbon dioxide retention associated with volatile anesthetics may also contribute to increases in ICP. Of the volatile anesthetics commonly used in veterinary medicine, halothane most dramatically inhibits the autoregulatory mechanisms controlling cerebral perfusion, increasing CBF and ICP [58]. Methoxyflurane, enflurane, and isoflurane interfere with autoregulation to a more limited extent [57]. Hyperventilation to reduce arterial carbon dioxide tension to approximately 30 mm Hg is rapidly effective in reducing CBF and ICP should either occur or in preventing their rise in at-risk patients. As such, modest hyperventilation should be incorporated into the anesthetic technique for animals in which autoregulation of CBF may be disrupted.

An anesthetic protocol has been suggested for horses with cervical stenotic myelopathy (CSM or wobbler's syndrome) and would seem to be appropriate for animals with SCI [57]. A low dose of xylazine (0.2–0.4 mg/kg administered intravenously) is used as premedication. The dose is minimized to avoid excessive ataxia. Anesthesia is induced using guaifenesin in combination with thiopental (5% guaifenesin with 0.3% thiopental) administered to effect. Alternatively, the guaifenesin may be administered alone until the horse becomes unsteady, followed by a bolus of thiopental (2–3 g per 450 kg of body weight). Anesthesia may be maintained with halothane, isoflurane, or injectable agents, such as guaifenesin and thiopental. Recovery from the guaifenesin and thiopental combination is generally relatively quick and acceptable if the duration of anesthesia is less than 1 hour. A low dose of xylazine (25–100 mg administered intravenously) is often given to ease recovery. Seizures in patients with spinal cord trauma should be treated initially with diazepam (0.03–0.1 mg/kg administered intravenously).

Airway management

It is clear from our understanding of the pathophysiology of SCI that maintenance of adequate oxygenation is critical in the initial management of these injuries. In adult equine patients with normally functioning lungs, arterial oxygenation may be optimized using intranasal oxygen insufflation at rates of 10 to 15 L/min [59]. Rates of 2 to 5 L/min are usually sufficient in foals.

Circulation

The acutely injured spinal cord is exquisitely sensitive to hypoperfusion. In human patients with SCI, early hypotension is associated with increased mortality and decreased neurologic recovery [60]. This is probably also relevant in equine patients with trauma, and vigorous volume resuscitation to normalize perfusion should be pursued. Unfortunately, SCI may impede this process with a loss of vascular tone and peripheral pooling of volume [8,9]. Additionally, sympathetic tone to the heart can be decreased, and unopposed parasympathetic drive may prevent reflex tachycardia or produce bradycardia. In these cases, central venous pressure monitoring may help to direct volume resuscitation [61]. Pressor therapy may be useful to reverse the drop in peripheral vascular resistance. In general, α-adrenergic agonists (eg, phenylephrine) are considered the most useful in human medicine [62]. Bradycardia may be treated with atropine or glycopyrrolate, although care must be taken to avoid gastrointestinal stasis in equine patients. In human clinical practice, mean arterial pressure targets of 90 to 100 mm Hg for 72 hours have been suggested, which requires strict attention to volume status and, in many cases, pressor therapy [54].

Treatment to prevent secondary injury to the spinal cord

Nonpenetrating wounds to the spinal column rarely result in complete transection of the cord, even in those individuals considered to have a functionally complete lesion [9]. Distal spinal cord function may be mediated by surprisingly small amounts of uninjured cord tissue, which is documented at less than 10% in some studies. Although perhaps on the horizon, there are currently no clinical techniques to restore neuronal losses after primary insult to the spinal cord. If some neural tissue survives the initial injury, however, interventions that limit the secondary pathophysiologic processes may improve the neurologic outcome. This type of neuroprotective treatment may be applicable to equine patients. The amount of normal spinal cord tissue required for acceptable function in equine patients is unknown and is influenced by anticipated future use. It is worth considering that only normal or near-normal neurologic function is acceptable in most equine patients. Furthermore, one should realize that months or years of intensive therapy and rehabilitation are required for many human victims of SCI.

There is a dearth of scientifically evaluated therapies for treatment of SCI in horses. In contrast, there is a huge volume of research on potential therapies in human fields. Unfortunately, many therapies that have seemed promising experimentally have been disappointing when applied clinically. The following is a brief discussion of a few of the more promising medical therapies that have been investigated in human medicine and may be applicable to equine patients. Surgical treatment has been described for some conditions of the equine spinal column and may be worth consideration, particularly in foals with minimal neurologic deficits [2,3].

Corticosteroids

The initial rationale for using corticosteroids to treat SCI was based on their ability to reduce cord edema [9,63]. The precise mechanism or mechanisms of action of corticosteroids are not fully understood but are thought to include the following: inhibition of lipid peroxidation, inhibition of the elaboration of inflammatory cytokines, modulation of cells of the immune system, improved vascular perfusion, and prevention of intracellular calcium accumulation [9,64]. A large number of animal studies have described improved outcome with corticosteroid therapy, although not all were able to demonstrate a beneficial effect [65]. Compared with other corticosteroids (eg, dexamethasone, hydrocortisone), methylprednisolone (MP) was thought to be superior for several reasons. Of the numerous mechanisms proposed for the beneficial effects of MP, the most important seems to be the drug's ability to inhibit lipid peroxidation [66].

Three large clinical trials (the National Acute Spinal Cord Injury Studies [NASCIS]) have claimed to demonstrate beneficial effects of MP treatment. These studies have been criticized, however, because of perceived problems in study design and statistical handling of the data. Post hoc analysis and arbitrary data stratification were necessary to obtain significant differences in outcome variables. Furthermore, the clinical significance of these differences has been questioned. Despite these concerns, MP may have some beneficial effects in a select group of patients when administered at extremely high doses (30-mg/kg bolus followed by a constant rate infusion of 5.4 mg/kg for 47 hours) within 8 hours of injury [9].

The National Association of Emergency Medical Service Physicians has recently published a position paper on the use of high-dose steroids for treatment of acute SCI [67]. This group contends that based on evidence from clinical trials, there is no indication that high-dose MP is effective in the treatment of acute SCI. Further, MP treatment is not without risk, and prolonged high-dose MP treatment seems to be associated with higher complication and death rates.

Opioid receptor antagonists

An increase in endogenous opioids occurs shortly after SCI, and the subsequent receptor activation is thought to be a contributor to secondary spinal cord damage. In some experimental models, treatment with the nonspecific opioid receptor antagonist naloxone reverses spinal shock and improves spinal cord blood flow (SCBF), with associated functional and electrophysiologic improvements [68]. These results have not been consistently reproduced, however. Naloxone comprised one of the treatment arms of the NASCIS II trial and was deemed to be of no value [69]; it has since been suggested that the dose used was subtherapeutic. Furthermore, re-evaluation of the data from that trial indicated that naloxone did promote motor and sensory recovery in patients with an incomplete SCI if given within 8 hours of injury [70]. More specific opioid receptor antagonists may also be beneficial in acute SCI. It has been shown that κ-receptor binding increases after SCI, and norbinaltorphinine (a κ-receptor antagonist) improved outcome in SCI in several rat studies [71]. The precise mechanism of action of the opioid antagonists is unclear.

Gangliosides

These are complex sialic acid–containing glycophospholipids present in high concentrations in cells of the CNS. They are located primarily within the outer leaflet of the lipid bilayer, forming a major component of the cell membrane [9,63].

Monsialotetrahexosylganglioside (GM-1 or Syngen) has been shown to accelerate neurite outgrowth and plasticity [72,73]. In addition, GM-1 prevents neuronal degeneration in some experimental models of CNS injury by attenuating excitatory amino acid release and inhibiting apoptosis [72,73]. In a large clinical trial, there seemed to be more rapid neurologic recovery in patients that received GM-1 [74]. Further, many parameters showed a trend toward improvement, particularly in patients with incomplete lesions. There was no difference in the primary outcome variable (proportion of patients achieving a marked recovery at 26 weeks after injury) in patients with complete paraplegia, however.

Thyrotropin-releasing hormone and thyrotropin-releasing hormone analogues

Thyrotropin-releasing hormone (TRH) is a tripeptide released from the hypothalamus that has several physiologic actions in addition to its hypophysiotropic role. TRH and its analogues may antagonize the action of some of the autodestructive factors within the CNS, such as endogenous opioids, platelet-activating factor, peptidoleukotrienes, and excitatory amino acids [65].

In animal studies, TRH significantly improved the long-term neurologic outcome, even if administration was delayed up to 1 week after injury [65,75]. In a small human trial, TRH resulted in a significant improvement in sensory and motor function 4 months after injury when administered within 12 hours of injury [76].

TRH analogues, which are resistant to enzymatic degradation and therefore have a longer half-life, have also been shown to be beneficial in experimental models [77]. In one series of studies, TRH or its analogues were found to be superior to several other treatments for SCI, including MP, dexamethasone, opioid receptor antagonists, calcium channel blockers, and serotonin receptor antagonists [76].

Antioxidants and free radical scavengers

Levels of endogenous antioxidants, such as α-tocopherol (vitamin E), retinoic acid (vitamin A), ascorbic acid (vitamin C), selenium, and certain ubiquinones (eg, coenzyme Q), are consumed after trauma [78]. Replacement of endogenous antioxidants may thus be effective in preventing damage caused by lipid peroxidation.

Pretreatment with vitamins A and C has shown benefit in experimental models of SCI [66,79]. Adequate levels must be available before injury, however, because CNS uptake is often slow (particularly for vitamin E), and clinical applicability may therefore be limited [80].

Several other compounds, including desferrioxamine, polyethylene-conjugated superoxide dismutase, and α-phenyl-n-tert-butylnitrone, have antioxidant properties or free radical scavenging ability and have shown benefit in experimentally induced SCI [63].

Sodium channel blockers

Local anesthetics, antiarrhythmic agents, and certain anticonvulsants that target sodium channels have shown neuroprotective effects in vitro and in vivo [9,63]. Sodium channel blockade with tetradoxin, although excessively toxic for clinical use, results in tissue sparing and improved functional outcomes after blunt trauma in experimentally induced SCI [81]. Studies examining other sodium channel blockers have also demonstrated efficacy. In a rodent SCI model, systemic administration of the sodium channel blocker riluzole provided significant neuroprotection, sparing gray and white matter [82]. Additionally, there was significant improvement in behavioral recovery after treatment. Riluzole has recently received US Food and Drug Administration (FDA) approval for treatment of amyotrophic lateral sclerosis (Lou Gehrig's disease). Human studies of this drug's application in SCI are not yet available, however.

Modulation of arachidonic acid metabolism

SCBF is maintained within normal limits after pretreatment with ibuprofen or meclofenamate in a feline SCI model. In the same study, pretreatment with a combination of a thromboxane A_2 inhibitor and prostacyclin analogue was also effective in limiting the decrease in SCBF [83]. The results of this and other studies demonstrate the importance of arachidonic acid metabolism in the regulation of SCBF. Prostacyclin, a natural end product of arachidonic acid metabolism produced predominantly by vascular endothelium, has potent vasodilatory activity and inhibits platelet aggregation. Prostacyclin derivatives and analogues, alone or in combination with mixed cyclooxygenase-lipoxygenase inhibitors, have shown benefits in models of SCI [84]. The expression of COX-2 has been observed to increase in the rat spinal cord after injury [34]. Specific inhibition of the COX-2 isoform was shown to improve functional outcome in moderately severe experimental spinal injuries [85,86].

Based on the importance of arachidonic acid metabolism in the pathogenesis of SCI, the widespread use of nonsteroidal anti-inflammatory drugs (NSAIDs) in the treatment of equine neurologic trauma is clearly justified. Specific COX-2 inhibitors are now available for veterinary use. Concerns have been raised regarding their safety and possible deleterious effects after treatment with these agents in veterinary patients, however [87].

Minocycline

Minocycline is a tetracycline derivative that is currently in common use for the treatment of acne and chronic periodontitis [44]. Minocycline has several neuroprotective properties, including inhibition of MMPs and microglial activation and reduction of neuroexcitotoxicity and apoptosis [44]. Several laboratories have reported improved functional outcome after minocycline treatment in models of SCI. As with many purported treatments for SCI, however, not all studies have found positive results, and some negative or even deleterious effects have been reported. A pilot study to evaluate minocycline in human patients has been initiated in Canada.

Immunosuppressive therapy

FK506 (tacrolimus) and cyclosporine are immunosuppressants that have demonstrated some beneficial effects in the treatment of peripheral nerve injury [88]. Cyclosporine acts at the mitochondrial membrane to prevent apoptosis. In SCI models, cyclosporine has been shown to promote tissue sparing and to inhibit lipid peroxidation. Similarly, FK506 has been shown to promote axonal regeneration within the CNS and to improve functional recovery after experimental SCI. FK506 has been approved by the FDA for the prevention of allograft rejection.

Erythropoietin

Erythropoietin (EPO) has been shown to have neuroprotective properties and to improve outcome in animal models of several neurologic conditions [44]. The hormone is thought to have anti-inflammatory, antioxidant, and antiapoptotic properties. In a small prospective study examining acute human stroke victims, EPO treatment improved neurologic function and reduced infarct size [89].

A potential side effect of EPO use is stimulation of erythropoiesis in nonanemic patients, which may lead to erythrocytosis and a prothrombotic state. It is possible that the molecule could be modified if the erythropoietic and tissue protective properties are mediated by different receptors and signaling pathways, however. In horses, recombinant human EPO (rhEPO) administrated as a performance enhancer has been associated with erythroid hypoplasia and anemia [90]. This was thought to be a result of anti-rhEPO antibodies that cross-reacted with the endogenous molecule.

Numerous other therapies for the treatment of SCI have been described, including the 21-aminosteroid (lazaroid) compounds, calcium channel blockers, and NMDA and AMPA and kainate receptor antagonists. Although these treatment modalities have a sound theoretic basis and have seemed promising in an experimental setting, they have been disappointing in clinical trials. This likely reflects the multifaceted nature of SCI and the many pathways involved in secondary injury processes. It is unlikely that single therapies are going to be wholly effective, and the search for appropriate combinations continues. For equine patients with SCI, practitioners should focus on rapid assessment, accurate diagnosis, and quality supportive care to limit further injury and optimize outcome.

References

[1] Jeffcott LB. Disorders of the thoracolumbar spine of the horse: a survey of 443 cases. Equine Vet J 1980;12:197–210.

[2] Nixon AJ. Fractures of the vertebrae. In: Nixon AJ, editor. Equine fracture repair. Philadelphia: WB Saunders; 1996. p. 299–312.

[3] Robertson JT, Samii V. Traumatic disorders of the spinal column. In: Auer JA, Stick JA, editors. Equine surgery. 3rd edition. Philadelphia: WB Saunders; 2005. p. 677–83.
[4] MacKay RJ. Brain injury after head trauma: pathophysiology, diagnosis, and treatment. Vet Clin North Am Equine Pract 2004;20(1):199–216.
[5] MacKay RJ. Peripheral nerve injury. In: Auer JA, Stick JA, editors. Equine surgery. 3rd edition. Philadelphia: WB Saunders; 2005. p. 684–91.
[6] McCue M, Davis EG, Rush BR. Diagnostic evaluation, clinical management, and transport of recumbent horses. Compendium on Continuing Education for the Practicing Veterinarian 2004;26:138–48.
[7] Davis EG, McCue M, Rush BR. Treatment and supportive care of recumbent horses. Compendium on Continuing Education for the Practicing Veterinarian 2004;26:67–77.
[8] Dumont RJ, Okonkwo DO, Verma S, et al. Acute spinal cord injury, part I: pathophysiologic mechanisms. Clin Neuropharmacol 2001;24(5):254–64.
[9] Kwon BK, Tetzlaff W, Grauer JN, et al. Pathophysiology and pharmacologic treatment of acute spinal cord injury. Spine J 2004;4:451–64.
[10] Wolman L. The disturbances of circulation in traumatic paraplegia in acute and late stages: a pathological study. Paraplegia 1965;2:213–26.
[11] Koyanagi I, Tator CH, Theriault E. Silicone rubber microangiography of acute spinal cord injury in the rat. Neurosurgery 1993;32(2):260–8.
[12] Tator CH, Fehlings MG. Review of the secondary injury theory of acute spinal cord trauma with emphasis on vascular mechanisms. J Neurosurg 1991;75(1):15–26.
[13] Blight AR, Young W. Central axons in injured cat spinal cord recover electrophysiological function following remyelination by Schwann cells. J Neurol Sci 1989;91(1–2):15–34.
[14] Senter HJ, Venes JL. Loss of autoregulation and posttraumatic ischemia following experimental spinal cord trauma. J Neurosurg 1979;50(2):198–206.
[15] Kobrine AI, Doyle TF, Martins AN. Autoregulation of spinal cord blood flow. Clin Neurosurg 1975;22:573–81.
[16] Guha A, Tator CH. Acute cardiovascular effects of experimental spinal cord injury. J Trauma 1988;28(4):481–90.
[17] Lukacova N, Halat G, Chavko M, et al. Ischemia-reperfusion injury in the spinal cord of rabbits strongly enhances lipid peroxidation and modifies phospholipid profiles. Neurochem Res 1996;21(8):869–73.
[18] McMichael M, Moore RM. Ischemia-reperfusion injury: pathophysiology. Journal of Veterinary Emergency and Critical Care 2004;14(4):231–41.
[19] Cuzzocrea S, Riley DP, Caputi AP, et al. Antioxidant therapy: a new pharmacological approach in shock, inflammation, and ischemia/reperfusion injury. Pharmacol Rev 2004; 53(1):135–59.
[20] Faden AI, Simon RP. A potential role for excitotoxins in the pathophysiology of spinal cord injury. Ann Neurol 1988;23(6):623–7.
[21] Choi DW. Excitotoxic cell death. J Neurobiol 1992;23(9):1261–76.
[22] Gasic GP, Hollmann M. Molecular neurobiology of glutamate receptors. Annu Rev Physiol 1992;54:507–36.
[23] Dawson VL, Dawson TM. Nitric oxide actions in neurochemistry. Neurochem Int 1996; 29(2):97–110.
[24] Mody I, MacDonald JF. NMDA receptor-dependent excitotoxicity: the role of intracellular Ca^{2+} release. Trends Pharmacol Sci 1995;16(10):356–9.
[25] Schanne FA, Kane AB, Young EE, et al. Calcium dependence of toxic cell death: a final common pathway. Science 1979;206(4419):700–2.
[26] Choi DW. Calcium-mediated neurotoxicity: relationship to specific channel types and role in ischemic damage. Trends Neurosci 1988;11(10):465–9.
[27] Faden AI, Chan PH, Longar S. Alterations in lipid metabolism, Na^+K^+-ATPase activity and tissue water content of spinal cord after experimental traumatic injury. J Neurochem 1987;48(6):1809–16.

[28] Eidelberg E, Sullivan J, Brigham A. Immediate consequences of spinal cord injury: possible role of potassium in axonal conduction block. Surg Neurol 1975;3: 317–21.
[29] Popovich PG, Wei P, Stokes BT. Cellular inflammatory response after spinal cord injury in Sprague-Dawley and Lewis rats. J Comp Neurol 1997;377(3):443–64.
[30] Dusart I, Schwab ME. Secondary cell death and the inflammatory reaction after dorsal hemisection of the rat spinal cord. Eur J Neurosci 1994;6(5):712–24.
[31] Bartholdi D, Schwab ME. Expression of pro-inflammatory cytokine and chemokine mRNA upon experimental cord injury in mouse: an in situ hybridization study. Eur J Neurosci 1997; 9(7):1422–38.
[32] Klusman I, Schwab ME. Effects of pro-inflammatory cytokines in experimental spinal cord injury. Brain Res 1997;762(1–2):173–84.
[33] Schwab JM, Brechtel K, Nguyen TD, et al. Persistent accumulation of cyclooxygenase-1 (COX-1) expressing microglia/macrophages and upregulation by endothelium following spinal cord injury. J Neuroimmunol 2000;111(1–2):122–30.
[34] Resnick DK, Graham SH, Dixon CE, et al. Role of cyclooxygenase 2 in acute spinal cord injury. J Neurotrauma 1998;15(12):1005–13.
[35] Kaufmann WE, Worley PF, Pegg J, et al. COX-2, a synaptically induced enzyme, is expressed by excitatory neurons at postsynaptic sites in rat cerebral cortex. Proc Natl Acad Sci U S A 1996;93:2317–21.
[36] Noble LJ, Donovan F, Igarashi T, et al. Matrix metalloproteinases limit functional recovery after spinal cord injury by modulation of early vascular events. J Neurosci 2002;22(17): 7526–35.
[37] Duchossoy Y, Arnaud S, Feldblum S. Matrix metalloproteinases: potential therapeutic target in spinal cord injury. Clin Chem Lab Med 2001;39(4):362–7.
[38] Levine JM, Ruaux CG, Bergman RL, et al. Matrix metalloproteinase-9 activity in cerebrospinal fluid and serum of dogs with acute spinal cord trauma from intervertebral disk disease. Am J Vet Res 2006;67(2):283–7.
[39] Emery E, Aldana P, Bunge MB, et al. Apoptosis after traumatic human spinal cord injury. J Neurosurg 1998;89(6):911–20.
[40] Crowe MJ, Bresnahan JC, Shuman SL, et al. Apoptosis and delayed degeneration after spinal cord injury in rats and monkeys. Nat Med 1997;3(1):73–6.
[41] Li GL, Farooque M, Holtz A, et al. Apoptosis of oligodendrocytes occurs long distances away from the primary injury after compression trauma to rat spinal cord. Acta Neuropathol (Berl) 1998;98(5):473–80.
[42] Eldadah BA, Faden AI. Caspase pathways, neuronal apoptosis, and CNS injury. J Neurotrauma 2000;17(10):811–29.
[43] Fiskum G. Mitochondrial participation in ischemic and traumatic neural cell death. J Neurotrauma 2000;17(10):843–55.
[44] Kwon BK, Fisher CG, Dvorak MF, et al. Strategies to promote neural repair and regeneration after spinal cord injury. Spine 2005;30(17S):S3–13.
[45] Deumens R, Koopmans GC, Joosten EAJ. Regeneration of descending axon tracts after spinal cord injury. Prog Neurobiol 2005;77:57–89.
[46] Licina P, Nowitzke AM. Approach and considerations regarding the patient with spinal injury. Injury 2005;36(Suppl 2):B2–12.
[47] Davis EG, Rush BR, McCue M. Equine recumbency: defining the problem and establishing the differential diagnosis. Compendium on Continuing Education for the Practicing Veterinarian 2004;26:67–77.
[48] De Lahunta A. Veterinary neuroanatomy and clinical neurology. 1st edition. Philadelphia: WB Saunders; 1977.
[49] Schott HC II, Carr EA, Patterson JS, et al. Urinary incontinence in 37 horses. In: Proceedings of the 50th Annual Convention of the American Association of Equine Practitioners. Denver (CO); 1985. p. 345–7.

[50] Schott HC II. Urinary incontinence and sabulous urolithiasis: chicken or egg? Equine Veterinary Education 2006;18(1):17–9.
[51] Gavin PR, Roberts GD, Papageorges M. The equine vertebral column. In: Thrall DE, editor. Textbook of veterinary diagnostic radiology. 3rd edition. Philadelphia: WB Saunders; 1998. p. 124–9.
[52] Kraft SL, Gavin P. Physical principles and technical considerations for equine computed tomography and magnetic resonance imaging. Vet Clin North Am Equine Pract 2001;17(1): 115–30.
[53] Bagley LJ. Imaging of spinal trauma. Radiol Clin North Am 2006;44:1–12.
[54] Chesnut RM. Management of brain and spine injuries. Crit Care Clin 2004;20:25–55.
[55] Available at: http://www.rescueglides.com. Accessed January 24, 2007.
[56] Moore RM, Trims CM. Effect of xylazine on cerebrospinal fluid pressure in conscious horses. Am J Vet Res 1992;53(9):1558–61.
[57] Harvey RC, Sims MH, Green SA. Neurologic disease. In: Thurman JC, Tranquilli WJ, Benson GJ, editors. Lumb and Jones' veterinary anesthesia. 3rd edition. Philadelphia: Lippincott, Williams, Wilkins; 1996. p. 775–85.
[58] Drummond JC, Todd MM. The response of the feline cerebral circulation to $PaCO_2$ during anesthesia with isoflurane and halothane and during sedation with nitrous oxide. Anesthesiology 1985;62(3):268–73.
[59] Wilson DV, Schott HC II, Robinson NE, et al. Response to nasopharyngeal oxygen administration in horses with lung disease. Equine Vet J 2006;38(3):219–23.
[60] Meguro K, Tator CH. Effect of multiple trauma on mortality and neurologic recovery after spinal cord or cauda equine injury. Neurol Med Chir (Tokyo) 1988;28(1):34–41.
[61] Magdesian KG. Monitoring the critically ill patient. Vet Clin North Am Equine Pract 2004; 20(1):11–40.
[62] Corley KTT. Inotropes and vasopressors in adults and foals. Vet Clin North Am Equine Pract 2004;20(1):77–106.
[63] Dumont RJ, Verma S, Okonkwo DO, et al. Acute spinal cord injury, part II: contemporary pharmacotherapy. Clin Neuropharmacol 2001;24(5):265–79.
[64] Gomes JA, Stevens RD, Lewin JJ, et al. Glucocorticoid therapy in neurologic critical care. Crit Care Med 2005;33(6):1214–24.
[65] Faden AI. Pharmacological treatment of central nervous system trauma. Pharmacol Toxicol 1996;78(1):12–7.
[66] Braughler JM. Lipid peroxidation-induced inhibition of gamma-aminobutyric acid uptake in rat brain synaptosomes: protection by glucocorticoids. J Neurochem 1985;44(4):1282–8.
[67] Bledsoe BE, Wesley AK, Salomone JP. High-dose steroids for acute spinal cord injury in emergency medical services. Prehosp Emerg Care 2004;8(3):313–6.
[68] Olsson Y, Sharma HS, Nyberg F, et al. The opioid receptor antagonist naloxone influences the pathophysiology of spinal cord injury. Prog Brain Res 1995;104:381–99.
[69] Bracken MB, Shepard MJ, Collins WF, et al. Methylprednisolone or naloxone treatment after acute spinal cord injury: 1-year follow-up data. Results of the second National Acute Spinal Cord Injury Study. J Neurosurg 1992;76(1):23–31.
[70] Bracken MB, Holford TR. Effects of timing of methylprednisolone or naloxone administration on recovery of segmental and long-tract neurologic function in NASCIS 2. J Neurosurg 1993;79(4):500–7.
[71] Faden AI, Takemori AE, Portoghese PS. Kappa-selective opiate antagonist norbinaltorphimine improves outcome after traumatic spinal cord injury in rats. Cent Nerv Syst Trauma 1987;4(4):227–37.
[72] Skaper SD, Leon A. Monosialogangliosides, neuroprotection, and neuronal repair processes. J Neurotrauma 1992;9(Suppl 2):S507–16.
[73] Ferrari G, Greene LA. Promotion of neuronal survival by GM1 ganglioside. Phenomenology and mechanism of action. Ann N Y Acad Sci 1998;845:263–73.

[74] Geisler FH, Coleman WP, Grieco G, et al. The Syngen Study Group. The Syngen multicenter acute spinal cord injury study. Spine 2001;26(Suppl 24):S87–96.
[75] Hashimoto T, Fukuda N. Effect of thyrotropin-releasing hormone on the neurologic impairment in rats with spinal cord injury: treatment starting 24 h and 7 days after injury. Eur J Pharmacol 1991;203(1):25–32.
[76] Pitts LH, Ross A, Chase GA, et al. Treatment with thyrotropin-releasing hormone (TRH) in patients with traumatic spinal cord injuries. J Neurotrauma 1995;12(3):235–43.
[77] Faden AI, Sacksen I, Noble LJ. Structure-activity relationships of TRH analogs in experimental spinal cord injury. Brain Res 1987;448(2):287–93.
[78] Rhoney DH, Luer MS, Hughes M, et al. New pharmacological approaches to acute spinal cord injury. Pharmacotherapy 1996;16(3):382–92.
[79] Anderson DK, Waters TR, Means ED. Pretreatment with alpha-tocopherol enhances neurologic recovery after experimental spinal cord compression injury. J Neurotrauma 1988; 5(1):61–8.
[80] Machlin LJ, Gabriel E. Kinetics of tissue alpha-tocopherol uptake and depletion after administration of high levels of vitamin E. Ann N Y Acad Sci 1982;393:48–60.
[81] Teng YD, Wrathall JR. Local blockade of sodium channels by tetrodotoxin ameliorates tissue loss and long-term functional deficits resulting from experimental spinal cord injury. J Neurosci 1997;17(11):4359–66.
[82] Schwartz G, Fehlings MG. Evaluation of the neuroprotective effects of sodium channel blockers after spinal cord injury: improved behavioral and neuroanatomical recovery with riluzole. J Neurosurg 2001;94(Suppl 2):245–56.
[83] Hall ED, Wolf DL. A pharmacological analysis of the pathophysiological mechanisms of posttraumatic spinal cord ischemia. J Neurosurg 1986;64(6):951–61.
[84] Hallenbeck JM, Jacobs TP, Faden AI. Combined PGI_2, indomethacin, and heparin improves neurologic recovery after spinal trauma in cats. J Neurosurg 1983;58(5):749–54.
[85] Lapchak PA, Araujo DM, Song D, et al. Neuroprotection by the selective cyclooxygenase-2 inhibitor SC-236 results in improvements in behavioral deficits induced by reversible spinal cord ischemia. Stroke 1983;32(5):1220–5.
[86] Hains BC, Yucra JA, Hulsebosch CE. Reduction of pathological and behavioral deficits following spinal cord contusion injury with a selective cyclooxygenase-2 inhibitor NS-398. J Neurotrauma 2001;18(4):409–23.
[87] Bertolini A, Ottani A, Sandrini M. Dual acting anti-inflammatory drugs: a reappraisal. Pharmacol Res 2001;44(6):437–50.
[88] Sosa I, Reyes O, Kuffler DP. Immunosuppressants: neuroprotection and promoting neurologic recovery following peripheral nerve and spinal cord lesions. Exp Neurol 2005;195:7–15.
[89] Ehrenreich H, Hasselblatt M, Dembowski C, et al. Erythropoietin therapy for acute stroke is both safe and beneficial. Mol Med 2002;8(8):495–505.
[90] Piercy RJ, Swardson CJ, Hinchcliff KW. Erythroid hypoplasia and anemia following administration of recombinant human erythropoietin to two horses. J Am Vet Med Assoc 1998; 212(2):244–7.

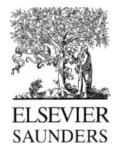

Injury to Synovial Structures

JoLynn Joyce, DVM

*Equine Lameness and Surgery, Department of Clinical Sciences,
Colorado State University, 300 West Drake Road,
Fort Collins, CO 80523, USA*

Wounds involving synovial structures, including joints, tendon sheaths, and bursae, are common injuries in horses [1]. The most commonly affected structures include the navicular bursae, distal and proximal interphalangeal joints, metacarpal or metatarsal phalangeal joint, digital tendon sheath, carpus, tarsocrural joint, calcaneal bursa, and tarsal sheath [1]. Knowledge of anatomy is important to confirm or rule out synovial involvement. Early intervention and treatment provide the best opportunity to reduce bacterial contamination and secondary long-term sequelae of synovial sepsis. Early recognition and intervention can often result in a good prognosis, whereas delayed treatment can result in life-threatening or career-ending conditions [2]. This article focuses primarily on synovial contamination by means of wounds and is intended to be a review of the diagnosis, pathogenesis of infection, treatment options, and prognosis of traumatic injuries to synovial structures. In general, septic arthritis and septic tenosynovitis are similar diseases and share similar clinical signs, diagnosis, and treatment. Individual and select cases are discussed.

Pathogenesis

Lower limb wounds are more likely to become infected as a result of environmental exposure and limited soft tissue coverage. Bacterial infection induces a synovial inflammatory response [3,4]. Neutrophils, monocytes, and other inflammatory mediators are attracted to the synovial space in an attempt to eliminate the infection [3,5]. As neutrophils phagocytize the foreign material, they release destructive enzymes and chemoattractants, such as collagenases, cytokines (interleukin [IL]-1), and tumor necrosis factor (TNF). This inflammatory response results in alterations in normal

E-mail address: jjoyce@colostate.edu

cell metabolism, reduced proteoglycan production, deposition of fibrin within the synovial space, and release of matrix metalloproteinases (MMPs) [3,5]. The physical effects on the synovial environment that occur as a result of this inflammatory reaction include increased intrasynovial pressure (puncture wounds), accumulation of fibrin (pannus), degradation of hyaluronan, and depletion of proteoglycans within the articular cartilage. As the duration of infection and inflammation becomes chronic, the synovial membrane may become hypertrophic; undergo vascular proliferation, thrombosis of synovial vessels, and pannus formation; and develop fibrosis of the joint capsule [1,6,7]. This can result in permanent damage to the synovial structure and cartilage.

Diagnosis

History and physical examination

An accurate history is important in determining the source and duration of the injury. Acute synovial wounds (<6–8 hours) may result in contamination of the synovial structure without developing a fulminant infection. Wounds introducing bacteria into a synovial structure for longer than 6 to 8 hours (chronic) have enough time to establish synovial infection (Fig. 1) [1,8]. These wounds present a treatment challenge. The prognosis depends on the ability to eliminate infection and effectively disrupt the inflammatory cycle that is harmful to bone, cartilage, and tendon [9]. The prognosis depends on the wound type, location, and longevity.

In acute injuries or in cases of large open wounds, the horse may initially show minimal lameness because of the lack of established intrasynovial

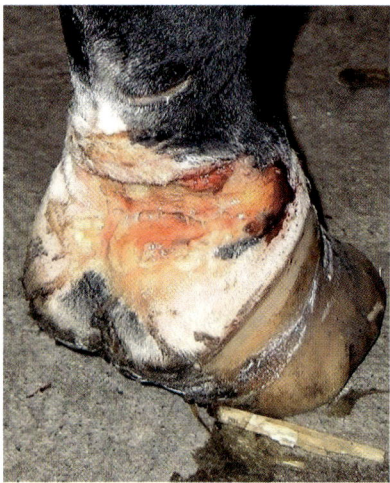

Fig. 1. Palmar pastern laceration extending into the digital tendon sheath resulted in severe lameness, continued drainage, and purulent exudate from the sheath.

pressure or inflammation. As untreated wounds become chronic, however, lameness can rapidly progress to severe and often results in poor weight bearing. Typically, the synovial structure (joint, tendon sheath, or bursa) has marked effusion with accompanying soft tissue heat, swelling, and pain on palpation and manipulation. Usually, vital signs are normal; however, tachycardia and tachypnea may be observed when horses are in extreme pain. The horse may or may not have leukocytosis and hyperfibrinogenemia and may or may not be depressed, febrile, and anorexic.

Wound preparation

When lacerations occur near a synovial structure, it is essential to determine if communication exists between the wound and surrounding joint, tendon sheath, or bursa. Before exploration of the wound, the wound edges should be clipped of all hair and debris using a sterile water-soluble lubricating gel (Surgilube Sterile Bacteriostatic lube) or a sterile saline–soaked gauze in the wound bed to prevent contaminates, such as dirt and hair, from entering the wound and to facilitate their removal. Strict aseptic technique should be used in all cases until synovial involvement can be ruled out. The wound should be aseptically cleaned with a combination of sterile saline (0.9% sodium chloride [NaCl]) and an antiseptic solution. Aggressive lavage with isotonic saline (0.9% NaCl) reduces bacterial numbers in wounds, with minimal adverse effects on tissues. Isotonic saline provides a fluid medium that neither causes cells to swell, as when using tap water, nor to crenate, as when using hypertonic solutions [2]. To be most effective at reducing bacterial numbers and removing foreign particles and devitalized tissue, irrigation should be delivered at greater than 8 psi and less than 15 psi. Several fluid pumps are available; however, a practical alternative to mechanical pumps is syringe irrigation. A 35-mL syringe and 19-gauge needle provide irrigant pressure of 8 psi and reduce surface bacterial counts 100-fold [10]. Once the wound is adequately cleaned, digital exploration (with sterile gloves) should be performed to determine potential structures involved (ie, exposed bone or joint, soft tissue involvement, presence of foreign material deeper in the wound). A sterile teat cannula or malleable probe is useful for exploration in puncture wounds and deep penetrating wounds to help determine the direction and depth of wound tracts.

Diagnostic modalities

If synovial involvement cannot be confirmed after digital exploration of the wound, several diagnostic modalities can be used to help confirm or rule out synovial penetration. It is important to obtain a synovial fluid sample in all cases of potential synovial penetration, because the synovial fluid analysis can aid in the diagnosis of sepsis and help to provide a therapeutic plan. The synoviocentesis (of a joint, sheath, or bursa) should be performed at a site distant from the wound in nontraumatized tissues. The area should be aseptically prepared and sampled. After collection of a sample, the needle should remain within the joint, sheath, or bursa and a large volume of saline (0.9% NaCl) or lactated Ringer's solution (LRS) should be infused into the synovial structure. If the structure holds pressure, it is likely not penetrated. If fluid exits the wound, however, synovial communication is confirmed. If the fluid collected grossly looks contaminated (cloudy, turbid), antibiotics should be infused before withdrawal of the needle. Antibiotics may be injected into the structure after distention.

Cytologic evaluation of synovial fluid samples is probably the single most useful test in evaluating a synovial structure with suspected infection [11]. Normal synovial fluid generally contains fewer than 500 nucleated cells/μL, with mononuclear cells being the predominant cell type (macrophages and lymphocytes) [11]. A total nucleated cell count exceeding 30,000 cells/μL and a total protein concentration greater than 4.0 g/dL with greater than 90% neutrophils are indicative of infection [12]. Infections within tendon sheaths and bursae may result in more variable changes in synovial fluid nucleated cell and total protein values (generally lower than those of joints) [1].

Radiographic evaluation of the affected structure is a useful means to obtain information, such as soft tissue swelling, presence of radiopaque foreign material, and fracture of surrounding bone. This is particularly important if there are lacerations to the calcaneal bursa and the tarsal sheath, wherein concurrent injury and osteomyelitis of the tuber calcanei and sustentaculum tali can develop. A flexed proximoplantar-to-distoplantar tangential (skyline) view of the tarsus should be taken to evaluate these areas. In chronic septic processes, radiographic evaluation may confirm or rule out concurrent osteomyelitis of the surrounding bone.

Contrast radiography can assist in diagnosis of synovial involvement. Navicular bursa penetration after a nail wound to the solar aspect of the foot may be difficult to determine by physical examination and plain radiography. Contrast radiography is helpful in determining wound involvement of tendon sheaths and other bursae (Fig. 2).

Ultrasonographic examination is a useful diagnostic modality, particularly in acute and chronic septic tenosynovitis. It can provide further evidence of sepsis by identifying excess fluid, fibrin formation, fibrous adhesion formation, and connective tissue integrity. Ultrasound may identify foreign material introduced by means of traumatic wounds. It may also guide fluid collection for synovial fluid analysis. Introduction of gas into deeper tissues may occur in acute traumatic wounds, limiting the effectiveness of this modality in these cases.

Therapeutic plan

Once synovial involvement has been confirmed, an appropriate therapeutic plan must be initiated. Factors that determine treatment of synovial injuries include duration of the wound, contamination of the wound, other

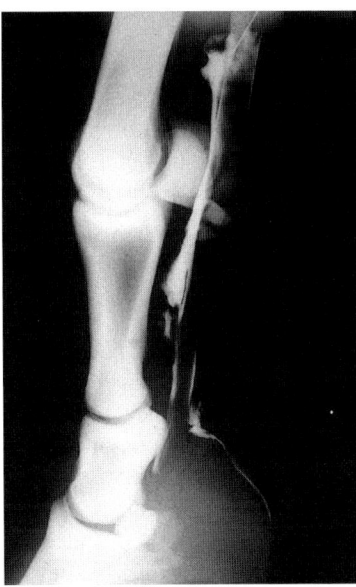

Fig. 2. Contrast material has been injected into the digital flexor tendon sheath and is exiting the wound at the level of the pastern, confirming penetration and communication with the tendon sheath.

structures involved, expectation of outcome and prognosis, and financial capabilities of owners. Treatment of septic arthritis or tenosynovitis is aimed at rapid elimination of the infection to minimize structural damage and fibrous adhesion formation [13]. The principles for treatment of infection for joints and tendon sheaths are similar; therefore, the following treatments are intended to apply to septic arthritis and tenosynovitis.

Identification of the causative organism(s) is important in the management of synovial infections. Although bacteria cannot always be isolated from synovial fluid, failure to isolate an organism from the synovial fluid does not rule out infection as the diagnosis [14]. It has been suggested that culturing the synovial membrane or fibrin results in greater probability of a positive culture. In one study in which synovial fluid and synovial membrane samples were submitted, however, growth was obtained from the synovial fluid in 16 (94%) of 17 joints, whereas growth was obtained from the synovial membrane alone in only 1 (6%) of 17 joints [11]. In general, infections that occur as a result of traumatic wounds generally tend to be polymicrobial because of environmental contaminates. In a retrospective study of 192 adult horses with septic arthritis or tenosynovitis, most of the bacterial isolates were aerobic and included Enterobacteriaceae, streptococci, staphylococci, other gram-negative and gram-positive bacteria, and miscellaneous isolates [15]. Another study found that *Staphylococcus aureus*, *Escherichia coli*, and *Pseudomonas aeruginosa* were the most commonly isolated organisms in horses with infectious arthritis [11]. Although a positive culture is beneficial in directing antimicrobial therapy, it should not be solely relied on for a definitive diagnosis. Regardless of whether a positive culture is obtained, if clinical evaluation, synovial fluid analysis, and other diagnostic tests suggest an infectious process, appropriate aggressive treatment must be implemented.

Systemic and local antimicrobial therapy

Systemic antimicrobial and anti-inflammatory therapy

Systemic antimicrobials are recommended for all horses with acute or chronic synovial injuries [1]. Although an appropriate antibiotic regimen can be implemented based on the results of culture and sensitivity testing of an organism, one should not prolong beginning antibiotic therapy while awaiting results. The horse should be placed on broad-spectrum antibiotics immediately after obtaining a synovial fluid sample for culture. Antimicrobials can be tailored based on the results of culture and sensitivity testing. The most commonly used drugs include penicillin (potassium penicillin, 22,000 U/kg administered intravenously every 6 hours or procaine penicillin G, 22,000 U/kg administered intramuscularly twice daily) combined with gentamicin (6.6 mg/kg administered intravenously every 24 hours). Other drugs or drug combinations, such as penicillin and amikacin (15–25 mg/kg administered intravenously every 24 hours); cefazolin (11 mg/kg administered every 8 hours); and gentamicin, ceftiofur (both administered intravenously or intramuscularly at a rate of 1 mg/lb twice daily), and enrofloxacin (5–7.5 mg/kg administered intravenously every 24 hours), can be used, however. In combination with other treatments (which are discussed elsewhere in this article), broad-spectrum parenteral (often intravenous) antibiotics are typically recommended for 7 to 10 days. If the horse is responding favorably, it may be switched to an oral antibiotic for an additional 2 to 4 weeks depending on the severity of the infection and wound and clinical progression. Typical oral antibiotics used include trimethoprim-sulfa, 960 mg (15 mg/lb administered twice daily); doxycycline, 100 mg (11 mg/kg administered twice daily); and enrofloxacin (7.5 mg/kg administered every 24 hours). In addition to systemic antimicrobials, horses may be placed on nonsteroidal anti-inflammatory medications. The typical drug of choice is phenylbutazone (2.2–4.4 mg/kg administered intravenously or orally daily). Other choices include flunixin meglumine (1.1–2.2 mg/kg administered intravenously or orally daily), ketoprofen (2.2 mg/kg administered intravenously daily), or carprofen (0.7 mg/kg administered orally daily).

Intra-articular or intrathecal antimicrobial therapy

Resolution of infection is improved when an appropriate antibiotic is delivered to infected tissues in concentrations greater than the minimum inhibitory concentration (MIC) [16]. Synovial vascular injury, ischemia, necrosis, and pannus formation can all occur in severe or chronic synovial wounds and markedly limit the delivery of systemically administered antibiotics to the synovial membrane. This limitation has led to the development of alternative techniques of antibiotic delivery. Intra-articular delivery of gentamicin was originally thought to be too irritating in equine joints [17]; however, it was later shown to cause minimal inflammation in normal equine joints [18]. Synovial fluid concentrations after a single intra-articular injection of gentamicin are 10 to 100 times greater than those achieved with intravenous administration [19], and *E coli* infection was effectively eliminated in an experimental model of septic arthritis using intra-articular therapy [20]. Based on these studies, intra-articular antibiotic treatment of synovial infections has become widely used. Intra-articular amikacin, an alternative aminoglycoside, has become a more favorable intra-articular drug because of its similar but broader spectrum of activity. The typical dose should not exceed the systemic dose, and the frequency of administration should be every 24 to 48 hours. When possible, the choice of antimicrobial should be based on cultured organism antibiograms.

Indwelling catheter and continuous intrasynovial antimicrobial infusion are current treatment modalities that can complement more commonly used treatments for septic arthritis or tenosynovitis. Placement of an ingress fenestrated drain in combination with open arthrotomy incisions allows daily lavage through the synovial cavity and administration of antibiotics [21]. In a recent study, a commercially available continuous infusion system (Joint Infusion System, Mila International, Florence, Kentucky) was used for intrasynovial antimicrobial delivery in horses with septic synovitis. The mean daily dose of gentamicin delivered by means of the infusion system was 1.8 mg/kg (0.08 mg/lb), and the mean daily dose of amikacin was 5.5 mg/kg (2.5 mg/lb) [22]. Intrasynovial levels of antimicrobials (gentamicin and amikacin) in this study were greater than 50 times the MIC for common equine pathogens, and 93% of synovial infections resolved [22]. In another study, a balloon constant rate infusion system (On-Q PainBuster post-op pain relief system; I-Flow Corporation, Lake Forest, CA) was used for delivery of antimicrobials in horses with septic arthritis, septic tenosynovitis, and contaminated synovial wounds. Each horse underwent synovial lavage with arthroscopic, tenoscopic, or through-and-through needle lavage, and the infusion system was placed at the time of lavage. A third-generation cephalosporin (2 g) or an aminoglycoside (2–3 g) was used to deliver an antimicrobial at a rate of approximately 100 mg/h. Thirteen of the available 16 horses for which follow-up was available were reportedly sound [23]. The use of intra-articular or intrathecal indwelling drains and constant infusion systems seems to be beneficial in treating synovial infections. They allow a simpler means of antimicrobial delivery and maintain high antimicrobial levels within the synovial structure. Additionally, they provide an opportunity for antimicrobial delivery in such locations as the stifles, elbows, and bicipital bursa, wherein regional limb perfusion has not been possible [22]. If an indwelling catheter or infusion system is used as an adjunctive treatment, it should always be treated in an aseptic manner and a sterile dressing should be maintained to limit ascending infection risk.

Regional limb perfusion

Regional intraosseous and intravenous limb perfusion techniques achieve high concentrations of antimicrobials in synovial fluid and bone and are effective in clinical and experimental infections [24,25]. Regional intravenous perfusion involves delivering an antibiotic under pressure to a selected region of the limb through the venous system [16], whereas regional intraosseous perfusion involves placement of a cannulated bone screw into the bone proximal to the infected synovial structure. Both techniques can be performed in an anesthetized or standing sedated horse by placing a tourniquet above the level of injury (or above the cannulated screw) for distal limb injuries or above and below the injury (for the carpus or hock). During intravenous perfusion, injection of a diluted antibiotic solution under pressure distends the venous vasculature and the increase in hydrostatic pressure allows diffusion throughout the tissues below or between the tourniquets [24,26]. It is performed by placing a small-gauge butterfly catheter or a small-gauge intra-arterial catheter into a vein and infusing the diluted solution of antimicrobial slowly over a period of 3 to 5 minutes. For both techniques, the tourniquet should remain in place for a 30-minute period to prevent systemic absorption of the drug, thus maximizing local tissue concentrations (Fig. 3) [1]. The typical antimicrobials and doses selected are similar to those previously described for intra-articular use and are diluted into 30 to 60 mL of sterile saline. In one study comparing intraosseous versus intravenous delivery of amikacin in equine tarsocrural joints, a greater concentration of amikacin was achieved in the synovial fluid after intravenous perfusion and was technically easier to perform [25]. Both techniques produced local antibiotic concentrations that exceeded the MIC for gentamicin and amikacin within the synovial fluid and bone, however [1,24–26].

Antimicrobial-impregnated polymethylmethacrylate

Polymethylmethacrylate (PMMA) is a high-density polymer formed by combining a fluid monomer and a powdered polymer. When an antimicrobial is added to this mixture, it becomes suspended in the polymer as it hardens [1,27]. The antibiotics incorporated in PMMA beads are released in a bimodal (rapid and slow) manner [21,27]. Rapid elution of the antimicrobial takes place, usually within the first 24 hours, and the subsequent elution rate is slower (weeks to months after implantation) [1,21,27]. This

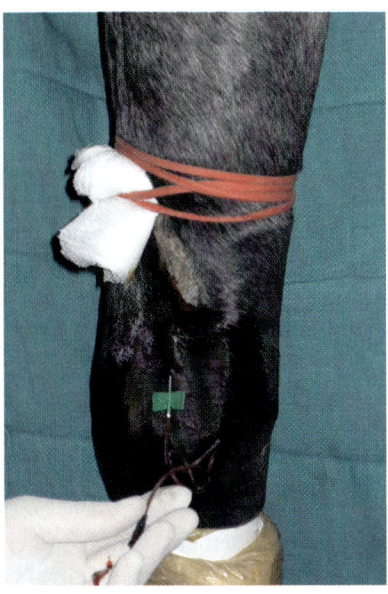

Fig. 3. Butterfly catheter is inserted into the cephalic vein for regional limb perfusion. The tourniquet is left in place for 30 minutes to allow adequate diffusion of antimicrobial to the wound in that region.

results in sustained release of antimicrobial compounds (up to 200 times that achieved through systemic administration) at the site of infection [1,27]. The antibiotic incorporated into the PMMA can be chosen based on the results of culture and sensitivity testing of the organism; however, it must be bactericidal, water soluble, and heat stable. Historically, powdered formulas were reported to be superior to liquid formulations; however, a more recent study has found that liquid antibiotic preparations are efficacious in PMMA [28]. Antibiotics that are most commonly used include gentamicin, amikacin, cefazolin, and tobramycin [1,21,27,29]. Typically, the concentration of antibiotic added to PMMA should approximate 5% of the weight of the PMMA (ie, amikacin, 0.5 g, for PMMA, 10 g) [21]. Because of their high concentration and prolonged release of antibiotics, antibiotic-impregnated PMMA beads may be a beneficial therapy in the treatment of infected synovial wounds. Long-term maintenance (9 days) of gentamicin-impregnated PMMA beads in the tarsocrural joint produced synovitis and superficial cartilage erosions [30]. Antibiotic-impregnated PMMA beads have mainly been advocated for use in orthopedic implant infections, long bone fractures, osteomyelitis, and soft tissue wounds. In the future, other biomaterials may be available that combine suitable elution characteristics in biodegradable or bioinert forms.

Synovial lavage and drainage

Physical removal of bacteria, inflammatory products, devitalized tissue, and debris is as important, if not more so, than antimicrobial therapy [3]. There are several techniques currently used to establish drainage and lavage of the synovial cavity. The aim of synovial lavage and drainage is to eliminate infection, and thus prevent damage to articular cartilage, and to reduce the formation of fibrous adhesions within synovial sheaths. Synovial lavage with a balanced polyionic electrolyte solution, combined with systemic and local antimicrobial therapy, produces the greatest chance for elimination of bacteria, resolution of infection, and return to soundness. Techniques most commonly used include arthroscopy or endoscopy, through-and-through lavage, and open drainage (arthrotomy). The technique chosen is directly related to the severity, duration, and location of the infection.

Arthroscopy or endoscopy

Endoscopic lavage and debridement is the preferred approach in all horses that have wounds with synovial involvement, especially in wounds greater than 24 hours old [1,31]. Arthroscopy, tenoscopy, and bursoscopy offer several advantages over other lavage techniques, including visibility of articular cartilage and related structures; guided removal of fibrin, debris, and osteomyelitic bone; and partial or complete synovectomy in chronic infections [32]. For these reasons, this technique has widely replaced through-and-through needle lavage in severe and chronic synovial infections. Endoscopic debridement and lavage has been shown to improve the prognosis for survival and to prevent loss of use in horses with contaminated and infected joints [3,31]. In a recent study in which endoscopy was used in conjunction with systemic and antimicrobial therapy to treat 70 horses with infected joints, 29 horses with infected tendon sheaths, 10 horses with infected bursae, and 12 horses with multiple infected synovial structures, 90% of these horses survived and 81% returned to their previous level of work [31].

Through-and-through lavage

Acute synovial injuries that are not significantly contaminated are appropriate candidates for through-and-through lavage. This technique is an inexpensive way of providing thorough lavage of synovial cavities. It is technically simpler than endoscopic surgery and can be performed multiple times in the standing sedated horse. Through-and-through lavage is performed by placing multiple large-bore needles (usually 14 gauge) or arthroscopic cannulas into the synovial space and infusing large quantities of fluid through the synovial space (Fig. 4). In one study of 15 horses that were presented within 2 days after an open joint injury, the mean number of joint lavages was 3.3 and the patient recovery rate was 87% [9]. In

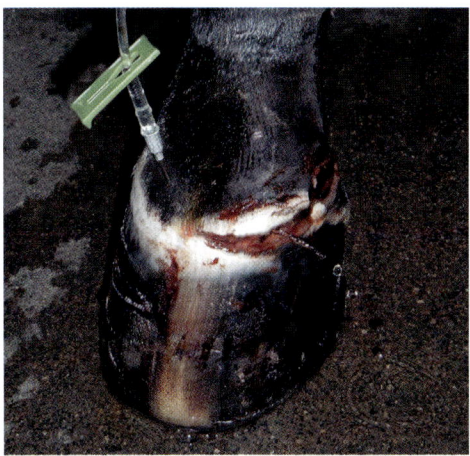

Fig. 4. This horse sustained a traumatic coronary band laceration communicating with the distal interphalangeal joint. An intra-articular 18-gauge needle has been placed, and through-and-through lavage of the coffin joint is being performed. The fluid is exiting readily from the wound.

more chronic cases of synovial injury, the efficacy of through-and-through lavage is lessened by the accumulation of fibrin, which obstructs flow through the needles. As discussed previously, in chronic synovial sepsis, endoscopic lavage is preferred because it allows removal of inflammatory debris and evaluation of the synovial structures.

Arthrotomy or ventral drainage

In chronic cases or cases that are refractory to multiple joint lavage or endoscopic debridement and lavage, open arthrotomy incisions may be beneficial to allow continuous egress of fluid and decompression of the synovial space. This is usually performed after endoscopic debridement and lavage, in which an incision is created at the ventral-most aspect of the synovial cavity to allow continued drainage of synovial fluid. This technique, combined with aggressive antibiotic therapy and joint lavage, was successful in resolving joint infection in 25 of 26 horses [13]. In this study, the arthrotomy incision needed to be debrided and closed in 9 horses, and no horses experienced desiccation of the articular cartilage or secondary infection of the joint by environmental bacteria [13].

Prognosis

The prognosis for horses that sustain traumatic injuries to synovial structures is influenced by the specific structure involved, duration of the infection before treatment, and presence of osseous or tendinous lesions

[1,31,33]. Multiple retrospective studies evaluating horses with traumatic synovial injuries have provided information on prognosis.

Septic arthritis

In one study evaluating open joint injuries in horses, 54% of horses treated survived long term [34]. Of 58 horses included in the study, 36 were euthanized for various reasons relating to poor prognosis, thus leaving 21 horses for which treatment was continued [34]. In the treated horses, the best outcomes and lowest infection rates were observed in horses that were treated by administration of antibiotics and surgical lavage and debridement within 24 hours of injury. In a similar retrospective study that included 192 horses affected with septic arthritis or tenosynovitis, there was an 85% success rate in adult horses that were treated aggressively for septic arthritis [14].

Septic tenosynovitis

The most common tendon sheath involved in synovial injuries is the digital flexor tendon sheath. Other tendon sheaths involved in lacerations include the tendon sheath of the extensor carpi radialis, the common digital extensor, and the tarsal sheath. Several retrospective studies have been performed evaluating the outcome of septic tenosynovitis in horses. In one study, 18 (78%) of 23 horses that were treated for septic tenosynovitis survived for longer than 6 months after discharge, with 10 horses (56%) returning to their previous level of performance [35]. Although there was no statistical difference between medical and surgical treatment, the authors strongly recommend treating all cases of septic tenosynovitis surgically for optimal results. In a more recent study, Frees and colleagues [36] reported that 18 (90%) of 20 horses survived and 14 (70%) returned to athletic soundness after tenoscopic treatment of contaminated and infected digital flexor tendon sheaths [32].

Septic bursae

A recent retrospective study evaluating septic calcaneal bursitis in horses reported a 67% survival rate, with 81% of those horses returning to full athletic performance. In this study, involvement of the tuber calcanei carried a guarded prognosis, with only 44% of horses in which this structure was involved surviving [33]. In a study of 16 horses sustaining penetrating wounds to the navicular bursa that were treated with endoscopy of the navicular bursa, 10 horses returned to their previous level of performance [37]. Endoscopic lavage and debridement is currently the treatment of choice for septic navicular bursitis. It allows the removal of fibrin and foreign material and the debridement of lesions on the palmar or plantar surface of the navicular bone and the deep digital flexor tendon. Endoscopic surgery has a lower morbidity rate than the streetnail procedure and improves the prognosis for horses with septic navicular bursitis [37].

Early studies of horses with synovial injuries revealed a fair prognosis for survival and return to function. More recently, the prognosis has improved, because early recognition and aggressive treatment increase our ability to treat many horses successfully. It is the author's opinion that early endoscopic surgical treatment, combined with systemic, intrasynovial, and intravenous regional perfusion of antimicrobials, is the most appropriate treatment for infected synovial structures and provides the most optimal results for return to athletic function.

References

[1] Baxter GM. Management of wounds involving synovial structures in horses. Clin Tech Equine Pract 2004;3:204–14.
[2] Hendrickson DA. Lacerations of synovial structures. In: Hendrikson DA, editor. Wound care management for the equine practitioner. Jackson (WY): Teton New Media; 2005. p. 173–8.
[3] Morton AJ. Diagnosis and treatment of septic arthritis. Vet Clin North Am Equine Pract 2005;21(3):627–49.
[4] Durham M, Dyson SJ. Applied anatomy of the musculoskeletal system. In: Ross, Dyson, editors. Diagnosis and management of lameness in the horse. Philadelphia: Saunders; 2003. p. 85–6.
[5] Bertone A. Infectious arthritis. In: McIlwraith C, Trotter G, editors. Joint disease in the horse. 1st edition. Philadelphia: WB Saunders; 1996. p. 397–409.
[6] MacDonald MH. The pathophysiology of equine synovial infections. Proceedings of American College of Veterinary Surgeons Veterinary Symposium 1995;5:43–6.
[7] Farstvedt E, Stashak TS, Othic A. Update on topical wound medications. Clin Tech Equine Pract 2004;3:164–72.
[8] Baxter GM. Management of wounds. In: Colahan PT, Mayhew IG, Merritt AM, et al, editors. Equine medicine and surgery, vol. II. 5th edition. Philadelphia: Mosby; 1999. p. 1808–27.
[9] Meijer MC, van Weeren PR, Rijkenhuizen AB. Clinical experiences of treating septic arthritis in the equine by repeated joint lavage: a series of 39 cases. J Vet Med A Physiol Pathol Clin Med 2000;47(6):351–65.
[10] Caron JP. Management of superficial wounds. In: Auer JA, Stick JA, editors. Equine surgery. 2nd edition. Philadelphia: Saunders; 1999. p. 129–40.
[11] Madison JB, Sommer M, Spencer PA. Relations among synovial membrane histopathologic findings, synovial fluid cytologic findings, and bacterial culture results in horses with suspected infectious arthritis: 64 cases (1979–1987). J Am Vet Med Assoc 1991;198:1655–61.
[12] Bertone AL. Infectious tenosynovitis. Vet Clin North Am Equine Pract 1995;11(2): 163–75.
[13] Schneider RK, Bramlage LR, Mecklenburg LM, et al. Open drainage, intra-articular and systemic antibiotics in the treatment of septic arthritis/tenosynovitis in horses. Equine Vet J 1992;24:443–9.
[14] Schneider RK, Bramlage LR, Moore RM, et al. A retrospective study of 192 horses affected with septic arthritis/tenosynovitis. Equine Vet J 1992;24:436–42.
[15] Moore RM, Schneider RK, Kowalski J, et al. Antimicrobial susceptibility of bacterial isolates from 233 horses with musculoskeletal infection during 1979–1989. Equine Vet J 1992;24(6):450–6.
[16] Whitehair KJ, Bowersock TL, Blevins WE, et al. Regional limb perfusion for antibiotic treatment of experimentally induced septic arthritis. Vet Surg 1992;21:367–73.

[17] McIlwraith CW. Treatment of infectious arthritis. Vet Clin North Am 1983;5:363–79.
[18] Stover SM, Pool RR. Effects of intra-articular gentamicin sulfate on normal equine synovial membrane. Am J Vet Res 1985;446:2485–91.
[19] Lloyd KCK, Stover SM, Pascoe JR, et al. Plasma and synovial fluid concentrations of gentamicin in horses after intra-articular administration of buffered and unbuffered gentamicin. Am J Vet Res 1988;49:644–9.
[20] Lloyd KCK, Stover SM, Pascoe JR, et al. Synovial fluid pH, cytological characteristics, and gentamicin concentration after intra-articular administration of the drug in an experimental model of infectious arthritis in horses. Am J Vet Res 1990;51:1363–9.
[21] Goodrich LR, Nixon AJ. Treatment options for osteomyelitis. Equine Vet J 2004;340–60.
[22] Lescun TB, Vasey JR, Ward MP, et al. Treatment with continuous intrasynovial antimicrobial infusion for septic synovitis in horses: 31 cases (2000-2003). J Am Vet Med Assoc 2006; 228:1922–9.
[23] Meagher DT, Latimer FG, Sutter WW, et al. Evaluation of a balloon constant rate infusion system for treatment of septic arthritis, septic tenosynovitis, and contaminated synovial wounds: 23 cases (2002–2005). J Am Vet Med Assoc 2006;228:1930–4.
[24] Mattson S, Boure L, Pearce S, et al. Intraosseous gentamicin perfusion of the distal metacarpus in standing horses. Vet Surg 2004;33:180–6.
[25] Scheuch BC, Van Hoogmoed LM, Wilson WD, et al. Comparison of intraosseous or intravenous infusion for delivery of amikacin sulfate to the tibiotarsal joint of horses. Am J Vet Res 2002;63(3):374–80.
[26] Werner LA, Hardy J, Bertone AL. Bone gentamicin concentration after intra-articular injection or regional intravenous perfusion in the horse. Vet Surg 2003;32:559–65.
[27] Sayegh AI, Moore RM. Polymethylmethacrylate beads for treating orthopedic infections. Compend Contin Educ Pract Vet 2003;25:788–94.
[28] Downes S. Methods for improving drug release from poly(methyl)methacrylate bone cement. Clin Mater 1991;7:227–31.
[29] Schneider RK. Orthopedic infections. In: Auer JA, Stick JA, editors. Equine surgery. 2nd edition. Philadelphia: Saunders; 1999. p. 727–36.
[30] Farnsworth KD, White NA, Robertson J. The effect of implanting gentamicin impregnated polymethylmethacrylate beads in the tarsocrural joint of the horse. Vet Surg 2001;30:126–31.
[31] Wright IM, Smith MR, Humphrey DJ, et al. Endoscopic surgery in the treatment of contaminated and infected synovial cavities. Equine Vet J 2003;35:613–9.
[32] McIlwraith CW, Nixon AJ, Wright IM, et al. Treatment of infection of joints, tendon sheaths and bursae. In: Diagnostic and surgical arthroscopy in the horse. 3rd edition. Philadelphia: Mosby; 2005. p. 427–39.
[33] Post EM, Singer ER, Clegg PD, et al. Retrospective study of 24 cases of septic calcaneal bursitis in the horse. Equine Vet J 2003;35(7):662–8.
[34] Gibson KT, McIlwraith CV, Turner AS, et al. Open joint injuries in horses: 58 cases (1980–1986). J Am Vet Med Assoc 1989;194:398–404.
[35] Honnas CM, Schumacher J, Cohen ND, et al. Septic tenosynovitis in horses: 25 cases (1983–1989). J Am Vet Med Assoc 1991;199:1616–22.
[36] Frees KE, Lillich JD, Gaughan EM, et al. Tenoscopic-assisted treatment of open digital flexor tendon sheath injuries in horses: 20 cases (1991–2001). J Am Vet Med Assoc 2002; 220:1823–7.
[37] Wright IM, Phillips TJ, Walmsley JP. Endoscopy of navicular bursa: a new technique for the treatment of contaminated and septic bursae. Equine Vet J 1999;31(1):5–11.

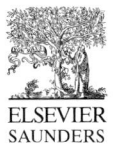

Field Fracture Management
Margaret C. Mudge, VMD[a],*, Lawrence R. Bramlage, DVM, MS[b]

[a] Equine Emergency and Critical Care, Department of Clinical Sciences,
The Ohio State University, School of Veterinary Medicine,
601 Vernon L. Tharp Street, Columbus, OH 43210, USA
[b] Rood & Riddle Equine Hospital, 2150 Georgetown Road,
Lexington, KY 40511, USA

Traumatic fractures, especially those involving the distal limb and skull, can be distressing to the horse and the owner. The initial management of fractures in the field is vital to the ultimate success of any repair, because stabilization and medical management are needed before referral for more definitive treatment. The principles of emergency first aid for equine patients with fractures have been delineated in multiple sources [1–5]. The emergency management of skull or facial fractures in the field has been addressed less extensively than the management of fractures of the appendicular skeleton, but many of the guidelines for client communication, patient assessment, and medical therapy are similar.

The general pertinent points of the physical examination, injury assessment, wound management, fluid therapy plan, pain management, and preparation for definitive treatment or referral are discussed. The specific methods of fracture stabilization or external coaptation as well as initial assessment of prognosis are more thoroughly covered in the sections on the individual fracture types.

General principles of medical stabilization of equine patients with fractures

Patient assessment

The initial assessment of a horse with a fracture of the skull or limb can present multiple challenges. Unstable limb fractures and displaced skull or facial fractures with significant hemorrhage can result in a horse with signs

* Corresponding author.
  E-mail address: mudge.3@osu.edu (M.C. Mudge).

of shock and an owner who is extremely anxious. Efficient and accurate assessment of the patient and adequate communication with the owner are fundamental to a successful outcome. Salient points in the physical examination include attitude, heart rate, mucous membrane color, capillary refill time, and an estimate of blood loss and other fluid losses (especially through sweating). Pale mucous membranes, prolonged capillary refill time, or significant tachycardia (heart rate >60 beats per minute) should signal a need for medical stabilization before referral. If there is ongoing blood loss or if the patient has an unstable limb fracture, measures to slow blood loss and to stabilize the fracture take priority over the medical examination outlined in this section.

Sedation and analgesia

Sedation is generally required for placement of limb splints or casts and may be required for diagnostics, such as radiography and endoscopy (in the case of a skull fracture). It is important to recognize signs of shock and hypovolemia in the patient, because these conditions may intensify the effects of sedation. Phenothiazine tranquilizers, such as acepromazine, should be avoided because they are likely to exacerbate hypotension attributable to α-adrenergic blockade and can cause fainting in excited horses [6]. Xylazine hydrogen chloride (HCl, 0.3–0.8 mg/kg administered intravenously) is useful for its sedative and analgesic properties, and at lower doses, it does not cause significant ataxia. Xylazine is relatively short acting (up to 30 minutes in duration); thus, longer acting α_2-agonists, such as detomidine (10–20 μg/kg administered intravenously) or romifidine (40–80 μg/kg administered intravenously), may be used if continued sedation is needed. Romifidine may cause less ataxia compared with detomidine, but the total dose is likely a greater factor than is the choice of sedative [7]. A twitch is useful to steady a fractious or anxious horse without contributing to ataxia.

Opioids and opioid agonist-antagonists can be valuable for additional sedation and analgesia in combination with the α_2-agonists. Butorphanol (0.01–0.04 mg/kg) and morphine (0.03–0.10 mg/kg) can be given intravenously in combination with α_2-agonists or can be given by the intramuscular route. Systemic opioids can be unpredictable when used without sedation; thus, they should be accompanied by tranquilization or sedation with an α_2-agonist. Although there are potential gastrointestinal side effects (ileus) associated with morphine and other opioids, morphine has not been shown to increase the risk of colic when used for perioperative analgesia [8].

Nonsteroidal anti-inflammatory drugs (NSAIDs) are still the mainstay of analgesic therapy in horses with musculoskeletal injuries. Phenylbutazone (2.2–4.4 mg/kg administered intravenously or orally), flunixin meglumine (1.1 mg/kg administered intravenously or orally), or ketoprofen (2.2 mg/kg administered intravenously) is an appropriate analgesic for patients with fractures. Fentanyl patches have been shown to be effective in combination with NSAIDs for treatment of pain in horses; however, adequate drug concentrations are not reached for approximately 14 hours [9]. Caudal epidural administration of opioids is not always practical for emergency pain management in the field but is a good option for hind limb and pelvic fractures. The use of local anesthetics, such as lidocaine, for epidural anesthesia is not recommended in patients with fractures because of the risk of ataxia. Analgesics should not pose a threat of further injury if the fracture is properly stabilized. Rigid stabilization should provide some relief of pain and anxiety, but analgesic medications are still indicated.

Anti-inflammatory medications

NSAIDs are the most commonly administered anti-inflammatory therapy for musculoskeletal injury in horses. Control of inflammation is an important step in limiting the risk of thrombosis, maximizing perfusion of the limb, and preparing the limb for surgical repair. Although corticosteroids are potent anti-inflammatories, their use is discouraged because of the risk of immunosuppression, possible potentiation of infection, and delay in fracture healing [10,11]. Dimethyl sulfoxide (DMSO) is a drug with anti-inflammatory properties that has been shown to reduce edema and scavenge free radicals. DMSO has been studied for use in treating inflammation and ischemia-reperfusion injury in horses with laminitis and large-colon volvulus; however, there is not strong evidence of efficacy [12,13]. Based on the theoretic and anecdotal benefits of DMSO, it would be most appropriate for injuries with severe soft tissue injury or devitalized tissue (0.1–1.0 g/kg administered intravenously), diluted to a concentration of 10%, given every 8 to 12 hours. The potential benefits include not only the possible anti-inflammatory effects but the increased perfusion of vascular-compromised tissue with antibiotic treatment. Mannitol (0.25–1.0 g/kg administered intravenously every 4–6 hours) can also be used to reduce edema and may be especially useful for patients with skull fractures at risk for cerebral edema [14]. Cold therapy and compression bandages are additional measures that can effectively reduce edema and inflammation.

Antibiotics and tetanus prophylaxis

If a wound is present over the fracture site, even if it does not seem to communicate with the site directly, the fracture should be considered open and appropriate antibiotic therapy should be initiated. Skull fractures that communicate with the oral cavity or sinuses are also considered open. A commonly used broad-spectrum combination is potassium penicillin (22,000 IU/kg administered intravenously every 6 hours) and gentamicin (6.6 mg/kg administered intravenously every 24 hours). Amikacin (21 mg/kg administered intravenously every 24 hours) can also be given in combination with a β-lactam antibiotic, such as penicillin, although its use is expensive in adult horses. Other antibiotics that could be considered are ampicillin, enrofloxacin, cefazolin, ceftiofur, and ceftazidime.

When there is an open wound associated with the fracture, tetanus prophylaxis should be considered. For horses with recent (less than 1 year before injury) tetanus vaccine status, a booster with tetanus toxoid can be given. If the horse's tetanus status is unknown or not up to date, a dose of tetanus antitoxin should be given (1500 IU administered intramuscularly).

Fluid therapy

Horses with distal limb fractures do not generally lose large volumes of blood; however, loss of blood, loss of fluid by means of sweating, and maldistribution of blood flow secondary to pain-induced vasoconstriction can result in shock [15]. Because packed cell volume (PCV) and total protein (TP) concentrations do not change immediately with acute hemorrhage and it is often not feasible to obtain blood work results rapidly in the field, measures of hypovolemia and shock must be made by careful physical examination (see section on patient assessment). Fluid resuscitation in the hypovolemic patient can be readily accomplished with intravenous crystalloids or colloids. Because the patient may be receiving potentially nephrotoxic drugs, such as NSAIDs and aminoglycosides, and may need to be trailered for several hours to a referral facility, fluid therapy in the field is often needed. As a general guideline for adult horses, lactated Ringer's solution or another balanced electrolyte solution should be given at a minimum dose of 10 L (20 mL/kg) to correct dehydration. The volume should be increased for patients that are showing signs of shock.

Neonatal foals have limited fluid and energy reserves; therefore, fluid therapy should not be neglected in these cases. If a foal has been unable to nurse because of a fractured limb, it may rapidly become dehydrated and hypoglycemic. A balanced electrolyte solution with dextrose (made to a 5% solution) can be used to replenish these deficiencies.

In the case of uncontrolled hemorrhage with nasal or frontal bone fractures or suspected large vessel laceration with femoral or pelvic fractures, the method of fluid resuscitation should be considered. A prospective trial in human patients with penetrating torso injuries showed an improved outcome in those patients who received delayed rather than immediate fluid resuscitation, sparking a debate over the timing and quantity of fluids to be administered in situations of uncontrolled hemorrhage [16]. We do not have evidence that the survival of horses with severe hemorrhage is improved with delayed or hypotensive resuscitation; however, controlled administration of fluids may be preferable to extremely large fluid boluses, which cause significant increases in blood pressure and may initiate more bleeding. If significant bleeding cannot be controlled, aminocaproic acid

(10–20 mg/kg administered intravenously, diluted in 0.9% saline [1–3 L]) can be given to inhibit fibrinolysis and stabilize the clot.

Prevention of thrombosis

Certain fracture types, such as fractures that disable the suspensory apparatus or fractures with severe soft tissue damage, are predisposed to vascular thrombosis. Any injury that causes severe stretch of the palmar or plantar vessels, even if the vessels are not ruptured, may lead to thrombosis, and successful fracture repair may not be possible. When vascular and severe soft tissue injuries are present with limb fractures in people, amputation rates can be as high as 61% [17]. Early initiation of systemic anticoagulant therapy in these injuries (when active hemorrhage is not present) has become the standard of care in human medicine and is recommended for equine fractures with significant vascular injury [17]. Aspirin (acetylsalicylic acid) has been shown to have antithrombotic actions in the horse at doses ranging from 10 to 20 mg/kg administered orally every other day [18,19]. Heparin has been recommended for prevention of venous thromboembolism in human patients and has been studied for use in the horse. Although low-molecular-weight heparin (LMWH) has been shown to have fewer side effects than unfractionated heparin in horses, LMWH is significantly more expensive [20]. Unfractionated sodium heparin should be given intravenously at a dose of 40–80 U/kg initially, and then at 40 U/kg subcutaneously every 8 to 12 hours. If calcium heparin is used, it should be given subcutaneously at a dose of 150 U/kg initially, then at 125 U/kg subcutaneously every 8 to 12 hours for 3 days, and then at 100 U/kg subcutaneously every 8 to 12 hours [21]. Protective external coaptation is especially important for fractures with vascular injury, because further motion and stretch can increase the risk of thrombosis. In the field, suspicion of vascular damage is based on skin temperature, pulse quality, and assessment of soft tissue damage or wound severity. Additional diagnostics, such as angiography and Doppler ultrasonography, can be performed at the referral facility if needed.

General principles of initial fracture assessment

Radiography

Unstable distal limb fractures must be stabilized before further diagnostics, such as radiography. Polyvinyl chloride (PVC) or wood splints permit diagnostic-quality radiographs with the splint in place, and this external coaptation can also help to relieve the patient's anxiety, further facilitating radiography. If a nondisplaced fracture is suspected and a radiographic diagnosis is not immediately available, appropriate stabilization should be applied based on the area of the limb involved (ie, do not wait for a radiographic diagnosis to stabilize the limb). Upper limb fractures can be difficult to diagnose with the equipment and facilities available in the field. The patient should not be anesthetized to facilitate radiographic diagnosis, because anesthetic recovery may cause a fracture to displace further. Rather, careful physical examination should guide medical stabilization and referral decisions.

Mandibular, maxillary, and frontal bone fractures can be imaged by radiography in the field, although careful palpation of the fracture is often revealing. Imaging of these fractures can be useful for detection of secondary problems, such as tooth root involvement, fluid in sinuses, and disruption of the calvarium.

Wound management

If the patient has an unstable fracture and is at significant risk of further soft tissue injury or fracture displacement, initial wound management may be minimal. In the case of the unstable limb fracture, proper coaptation of the limb has the first priority. The limb should be cleaned of any gross contamination, and any open wounds should be covered with a water-soluble antibiotic ointment and bandaged to minimize exposure of the tissues to ambient bacteria. Even if the skin is not broken, the area over the fracture should be cleaned and bandaged to prevent potential contamination if the fracture should become open.

Prognosis

Despite significant advances in fracture repair, open and severely displaced long bone fractures in adult horses still have a grave prognosis. Open fractures of the radius and tibia, in particular, have a poor prognosis. The weight and temperament of the horse can also factor into the prognosis, with lighter horses (<400–600 lb) and those with a calm temperament having a better prognosis [5]. The prognosis should be discussed with the owner, and accurate information should be gathered from the referral center so that an informed decision can be made regarding referral for fracture fixation. Many fractures that have a guarded prognosis in adult horses actually have a good prognosis with surgical fixation in foals.

Fractures of the appendicular skeleton

Principles of fracture stabilization

The goals of fracture stabilization are to prevent further injury to bone and soft tissue and to help assist weight bearing and relieve anxiety in the horse. All fractures should be protected from forces that tend to displace the fracture, and closed fractures should be protected against becoming open. The ideal splint should also protect the soft tissues, including vessels and nerves, from further trauma. Fracture instability can lead to severely damaged surrounding soft tissue, disrupted blood supply, or eburnated bone ends, resulting in a worsened prognosis.

A variety of splints or casts can be used to stabilize fractures of the distal limb. The ideal splint should be rigid, lightweight, and easily applied under standing sedation. PVC splints are effective for a variety of fractures, and splints of varying lengths can be cut ahead of time for use in emergencies. If a PVC splint is not available, a wooden board, broom handle, or metal rod can also be used to provide rigid coaptation. When the splint is applied over a bandage, nonelastic tape should be used to secure the splint; elastic tape allows the splint to slip and may cause more damage to the fractured limb. Fiberglass casting tape (VetCast; 3M, St. Paul, Minnesota) adds strength and rigidity to the external coaptation, but casting material may not be effectively applied if there is too much motion at the fracture site or if the patient is not sufficiently tractable. In addition to the splint or cast constructions, there are a variety of commercially available splints that can be used for distal limb fractures.

The forelimb and hind limb can be divided into four regions for the purposes of guidelines for application of external stabilization [1]. The limb divisions are as follows: (1) distal to distal metacarpus or metatarsus, (2) distal radius to distal metacarpus or proximal metatarsus to distal metatarsus, (3) elbow to distal radius or stifle to proximal metatarsus, and (4) proximal to elbow joint or stifle joint (Fig. 1). These divisions

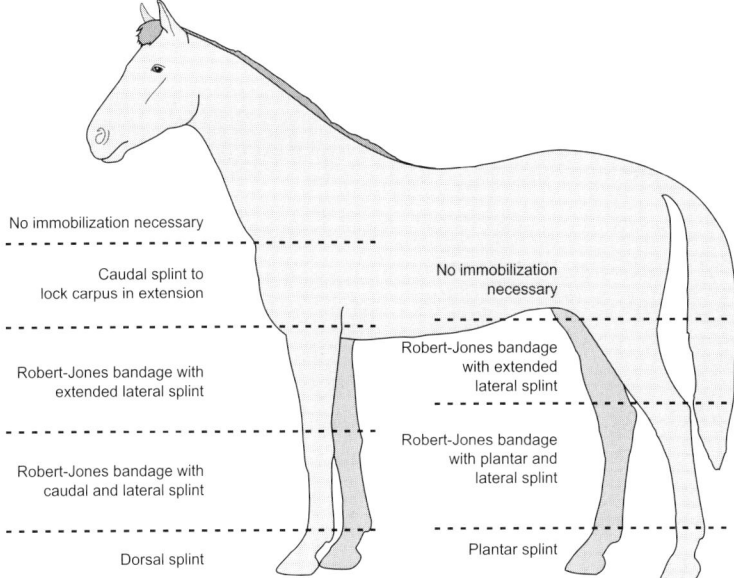

Fig. 1. Functional divisions for external coaptation of limb fractures. (*Adapted from* Bramlage LR. First aid and transportation of fracture patients. In: Nixon AJ, editor. Equine fracture repair. Philadelphia: WB Saunders; 1996. p. 38; with permission.)

can be used to guide stabilization of fractures, luxations, or severe lacerations. Recommendations for specific fracture types are described in the next sections.

Distal limb (first and second phalanges, proximal sesamoid bones)

When a distal limb fracture occurs and the fetlock is in the normal anatomic position, the primary bending force becomes the fracture site rather than the fetlock joint [1]. Neutralization of this bending force can be accomplished by splinting or casting the patient, with the dorsal cortices of the bones (metacarpal or metatarsal, P1, P2, and P3) in alignment (Fig. 2). For the forelimb, the splint is placed over a light bandage on the dorsal aspect of the limb. A plantar splint is placed for hind limb fractures (Fig. 3). The splint can be strengthened with the addition of fiberglass casting material, and a heel wedge or casting material placed under the heel can help to stabilize the limb in rigid alignment. There are several commercially available splints that are suitable for distal limb (level 1) fractures. The commercially available Leg Saver splint (Kimzey, Woodland, California) can be readily applied in the field, although it does not provide medial-to-lateral stability and does not accommodate large feet. The "Straight to the Toe" brace can also be used for stabilization of distal

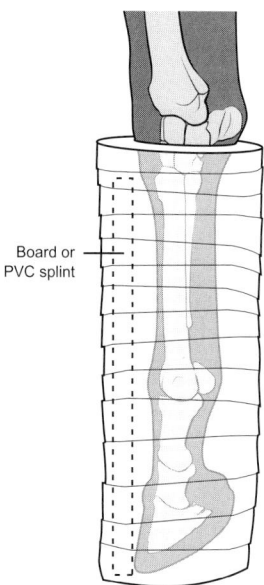

Fig. 2. Dorsal splint to prevent fetlock bending forces in distal limb fractures (forelimb). (*Adapted from* Bramlage LR. First aid and transportation of fracture patients. In: Nixon AJ, editor. Equine fracture repair. Philadelphia: WB Saunders; 1996. p. 38; with permission.)

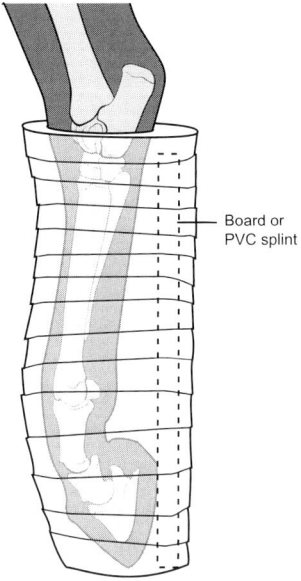

Fig. 3. Plantar splint for stabilization of level 1 fractures of the hind limb. (*Adapted from* Bramlage LR. First aid and transportation of fracture patients. In: Nixon AJ, editor. Equine fracture repair. Philadelphia: WB Saunders; 1996. p. 40; with permission.)

limb fractures (Equine Bracing Solutions, Trumansburg, New York, available at: http://www.equinebracing.com).

Distal metacarpal or metatarsal condyle

Fractures of the distal condyle of the metacarpus or metatarsus are relatively common injuries in the racehorse population and have a good prognosis, provided that significant displacement of the fracture is avoided and the soft tissues are adequately protected [22,23]. Because only a portion of the distal metacarpus is fractured, these fractures do not tend to be as unstable in bending (flexion or extension of the fetlock) as do fractures of P1 and P2, but they do require some medial-to-lateral support. Incomplete or nondisplaced fractures can be managed in a simple distal limb bandage while awaiting further diagnosis or definitive treatment. Displaced fractures of the distal condyle can be stabilized in a distal limb cast with the limb in neutral position, or they can be stabilized in a commercially available splint or cast that provides circumferential support (Fetlock Stabilizing Brace; Equine Bracing Solutions). The Leg Saver splint, although suitable for P1 and P2 fractures as well as for flexor tendon lacerations and some suspensory ligament injuries, is not ideal for condylar fractures because it does not provide medial-to-lateral support.

Condylar fractures in combination with distal sesamoidean ligament avulsion or bilateral proximal sesamoid bone fractures ("break down injury") require coaptation that prevents hyperextension of the fetlock as well as providing medial-to-lateral support. A splint, cast, or commercially available brace that aligns the dorsal cortices of the phalanges and metacarpus or metatarsus is needed to stabilize these injuries. Injuries that allow hyperextension of the fetlock put the patient at risk of significant vascular injury attributable to repeated stretching of the vessels; thus, anti-inflammatory and antithrombotic medications should be initiated.

Midforelimb or middle hind limb (mid- to proximal metacarpus or tarsus, carpus, distal radius)

Fractures of the midforelimb (level 2) require rigid stabilization with splints placed at 90° angles, extending from the elbow to the ground. A Robert Jones bandage should be placed first, using multiple layers of cotton padding with elastic gauze to compress each layer and building to a diameter approximately three times the diameter of the limb at the fracture site. For fractures of the forelimb, the splints should be applied caudally and laterally, extending from the elbow to the ground. The splint can be reinforced with fiberglass casting material for added rigidity. For hind limb fractures, fewer layers of bandage material are placed and the caudal splint can extend only to the level of the calcaneus because of the angulation of the hock. The lateral splint can be extended to the level of the stifle (especially for fractures of the proximal metatarsus).

Olecranon

The ulna is not a weight-bearing bone, and stabilization is neither as difficult nor as critical as for a radius fracture. The primary force on the ulna is the pull of the triceps muscle. When a complete fracture occurs, the function of the triceps muscle is disrupted and the horse can no longer keep the limb in extension. This loss of triceps action can result in significant distress or anxiety to the horse, because it is difficult to use the limb for support even when standing. These horses have a typical "dropped elbow" appearance and tend to buckle at the carpus when they attempt to bear weight. A full-limb bandage with caudal and lateral splints or an extended lateral splint is unnecessary in these cases. A caudal splint that keeps the carpus in extension is generally sufficient to allow weight bearing (Fig. 4). This type of splint is also useful for patients with radial nerve paralysis or for patients with humeral fractures that have lost triceps muscle function.

Mid- and proximal radius

When there is an unstable fracture of the radius, the force generated by the flexor and extensor muscles is altered. These muscles act primarily as

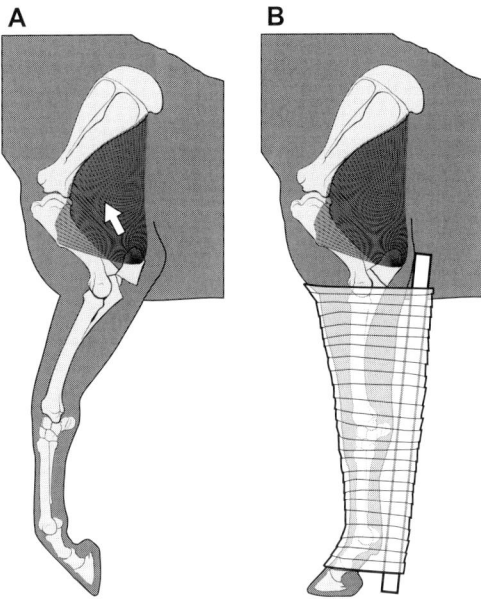

Fig. 4. Lateral splint for stabilization of a mid-to-proximal radius fracture. (*A*) Abduction of the limb results in fracture displacement through the thin skin at the medial aspect of the limb. (*B*) Robert Jones bandage with extended lateral splint prevents abduction of the limb. (*Adapted from* Fürst AE. Emergency treatment and transportation of equine fracture patients. In: Auer JA, Stick JA, editors. Equine surgery. 3rd edition. St. Louis (MO): WB Saunders; 2006. p. 977; with permission.)

abductors because of their lateral position in relation to the fractured bone, potentially causing a closed fracture to become open through the thin medial skin covering. A Robert Jones bandage with caudal and lateral splints, similar to that utilized for a proximal metacarpal fracture, is used to stabilize the fracture. To counteract abductor forces, the lateral splint is extended to the level of the shoulder and taped securely at the axilla so that contact with the shoulder prevents limb abduction (Fig. 5).

Tibia

Similar to the forces on the radius after a complete fracture, the extensors of the hind limb act as abductors and tend to cause further displacement and overriding of the tibial fracture. Because the stifle cannot be immobilized, the reciprocal apparatus acts to cause further overriding of the fracture. A lateral splint extended to the level of the hip does offer protection against abduction and displacement through the thin medial skin over the tibia. Because of the angle of the hock, it is difficult to achieve rigid stabilization with a splint. A straight, flat, and wide board that spans the hock and stifle

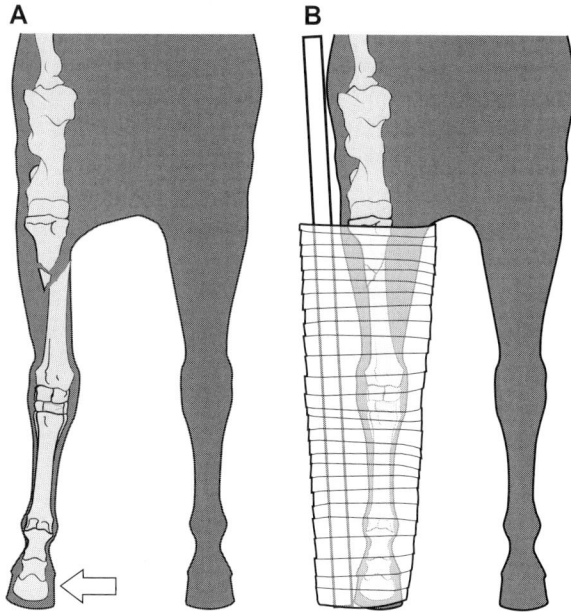

Fig. 5. (*A*) Complete olecranon fracture results in disruption of the triceps apparatus. (*B*) Caudal splint stabilizes the carpus in extension and allows weight bearing. (*Adapted from* Fürst AE. Emergency treatment and transportation of equine fracture patients. In: Auer JA, Stick JA, editors. Equine surgery. 3rd edition. St. Louis (MO): WB Saunders; 2006. p. 977; with permission.)

joints or an angled splint makes the limb less likely to rotate and the splint less likely to displace (Fig. 6).

Humerus or femur and above this level

The musculature of the upper limb and shoulder adequately stabilizes many fractures of the humerus and scapula. Attempts to splint these fractures may create more distraction of the fracture because of the weight of the splint. The patient may not be able to lock the carpus in extension with a fracture of the humerus, especially in combination with damage to the radial nerve. A light caudal splint that fixes the carpus in extension can be useful in these cases. Referral for internal fixation is indicated for foals with fractures of the humerus; however, adult horses may have a successful outcome with conservative management [24].

Fractures of the femur and pelvis also cannot be stabilized by external coaptation, and splinting should not be attempted. A lightweight compression bandage can prevent the distal limb edema that often occurs secondary to the upper limb fracture. Femoral fractures and pelvic fractures have been associated with significant hemorrhage; thus, these patients should be evaluated carefully for signs of hemorrhage and should be moved minimally

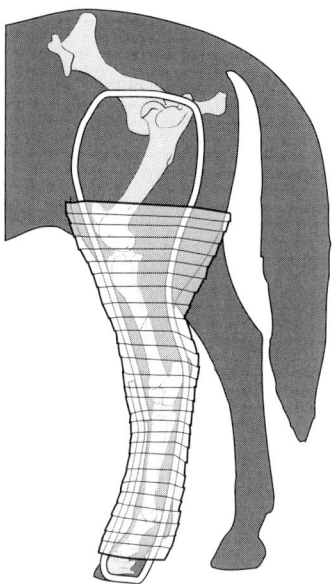

Fig. 6. Lateral hind limb splint appropriate for stabilization of tibial fractures.

[25–27]. Successful conservative management has been reported for pelvic fractures [27,28]. Conservative management has also been successful for the treatment of femoral fractures, but foals should be referred for surgical repair to avoid angular limb deformity in the contralateral limb [29].

Fractures of the skull, mandible, and maxilla

Although rarely life threatening, fractures of the maxilla, mandible, nasal, and frontal bones can have a dramatic appearance and can be associated with significant hemorrhage and respiratory compromise. Any horse with a traumatic skull fracture should be examined for signs of significant hemorrhage, respiratory compromise, neurologic deficits, and periocular or ocular involvement (neurologic and ophthalmic sequelae are addressed in other articles in this issue).

Mandibular and premaxillary fractures

Fractures of the rostral mandible, incisors, and premaxilla are usually readily evident on physical examination and palpation. Radiographs, especially intraoral views, can be helpful to determine the exact fracture configuration and any tooth involvement. Bilateral mandibular fractures tend to result in protrusion of the tongue and difficulty in prehension of food. Significant blood and salivary losses, combined with decreased water consumption, can lead to dehydration; thus, fluid therapy is often indicated. Although these fractures do not require emergency stabilization for a successful outcome, early repair can increase the horse's comfort and increase its willingness to eat and drink. Unilateral fractures may be managed without fixation, but bilateral fractures should be repaired. Simple incisor fractures may be repaired by intraoral wire fixation, and if the horse is amenable, this repair can be accomplished under standing sedation with local anesthesia of the mental or infraorbital nerves (Fig. 7). More complex fractures require referral for intraoral splinting, external skeletal fixation, dynamic compression plating, or lag screw fixation [30,31]. If the horse is at risk of further traumatizing the mandible or maxilla, a muzzle can be placed until definitive repair is accomplished.

Nasal, frontal, and maxillary bone fractures

The nasal and frontal bones are extremely vascular structures, and hemorrhage can be significant even with less severe fractures. The owner may report considerable bleeding, but a physical examination and serial PCV and TP measurements can more clearly define the severity of blood loss. Although many skull and sinus fractures do not require immediate treatment, severe hemorrhage, ocular involvement, respiratory compromise, and neurologic deficits do require emergency treatment or stabilization. Depression fractures that partially occlude the nasal passages may cause respiratory difficulty. Endoscopy of the upper aiways can aid in defining the obstruction and locating the source of bleeding. In cases of significant respiratory distress, an emergency tracheostomy can be performed before

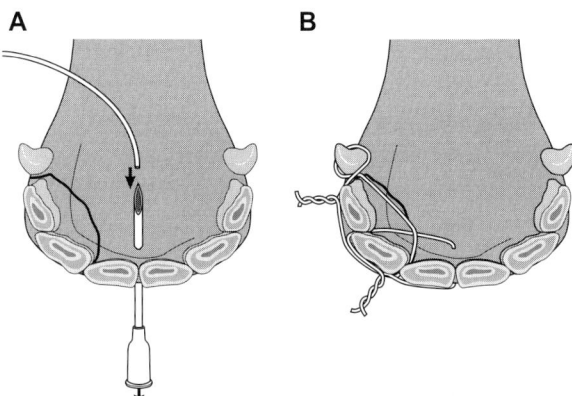

Fig. 7. Cerclage wiring of an incisor fracture. (*A*) Fourteen-gauge needle is used to guide 1.25-mm stainless-steel wire between incisors. (*B*) Cerclage loops stabilize the fracture using the adjacent incisor and the adjacent canine tooth. (*Adapted from* Auer JA. Craniomaxillofacial disorders. In: Auer JA, Stick JA, editors. Equine surgery. 3rd edition. St. Louis (MO): WB Saunders; 2006. p. 1344; with permission.)

further diagnostics. The fracture should be considered open if there is any disruption of the nasal or sinus mucosa. If surgical repair is planned or there is significant bleeding into the sinuses, broad-spectrum antibiotics should be administered. Sinus lavage can also be performed to reduce the risk of sinus empyema. Lavage can be performed in the field by creating a portal in the frontal sinus with a 6-mm Steinmann pin and infusing 0.9% saline or lactated Ringer's solution [30].

Depression fractures that are stable and do not interfere with the orbit or the airway may be treated conservatively. Fractures of the skull tend to heal quickly because of good blood supply and minimal loading forces. Conservative management of skull or facial fractures may result in cosmetic blemish, or possibly, callus that interferes with air flow or sinus drainage. If surgical repair is planned, medical treatment to reduce inflammation and edema of the soft tissues can aid in identification of landmarks and manipulation during surgery.

Transportation of equine patients with fractures

Even when properly stabilized, many long bone fractures still incur further damage, especially during transportation. Ideally, the trailer should have a loading ramp so that the horse does not have to step up. Nonslip floors are ideal, but shavings can be added to the trailer floor to provide better footing. It is important that the horse be confined to a small area with partitions and chest bars so that it can use these supports to maintain its balance during transportation. It is easier to control acceleration than it is to control braking; thus, when feasible, horses with forelimb fractures should be faced backward in the trailer so that their weight is thrown onto the hind limbs during braking. Similarly, horses with hind limb fractures should be positioned facing forward in the trailer. Although maintaining balance is more easily accomplished in these positions, unloading the horse from the trailer may be more difficult when the injured limb must come off first. A large van can allow the horse to be maneuvered so that the sound limbs exit the trailer first. Custom emergency trailers can be equipped with a harness system that can support the injured horse and prevent excessive distress or weight bearing on the injured limb [4]. Foals may be transported separated from the dam and, ideally, with an attendant. If an attendant is available, foals may be sedated or lightly anesthetized so that they do not struggle during transport.

Although it is generally not possible to stabilize skull fractures for transport, a head protector can be used to help prevent further soft tissue damage or trauma (Equine head protector; Jupiter Veterinary Products, Harrisburg, Pennsylvania). For horses with fractures involving the orbit or periorbital region, a hood with a protective ball cup can be used to protect the eye (EyeSaver; Jupiter Veterinary Products).

Summary

The management of equine fractures in the field begins with careful assessment of the fracture as well as the metabolic status of the patient. Proper stabilization of the fracture is essential to a successful outcome, and an improperly placed splint can cause significant soft tissue damage or worsening of the fracture. Although fracture stabilization and, ultimately, surgical repair of the fracture are central components of fracture management, the medical treatment of the patient also plays a key role in the morbidity and mortality of these cases. Advances in pain management, fluid resuscitation protocols, antithrombotic medications, and emergency transportation vehicles have increased our ability to stabilize horses before definitive treatment of the fracture.

References

[1] Bramlage LR. Current concepts of emergency first aid treatment and transportation of equine fracture patients. Compendium on Continuing Education for the Practicing Veterinarian 1983;5(10):S564–73.
[2] Bramlage LR. First aid and transportation of fracture patients. In: Nixon AJ, editor. Equine fracture repair. Philadelphia: WB Saunders; 1996. p. 36–42.
[3] Bertone AL. Management of orthopedic emergencies. Vet Clin North Am Equine Pract 1994;10(3):603–25.
[4] Fürst AE. Emergency treatment and transportation of equine fracture patients. In: Auer JA, Stick JA, editors. Equine surgery. 3rd edition. St. Louis (MO): Saunders; 2006. p. 972–81.
[5] McIlwraith CW, Orsini JA. Musculoskeletal system. In: Orsini JA, Divers TJ, editors. Manual of equine emergencies. 2nd edition. Philadelphia: Mosby; 2003. p. 343–87.
[6] Muir WW, Hubbell JAE, Skarda RT, et al, editors. Handbook of veterinary analgesia. 3rd edition. St. Louis (MO): 2000. p. 19–40.
[7] Figueiredo JP, Muir WW, Smith J, et al. Sedative and analgesic effects of romifidine in horses. Intern J Appl Res Vet Med 2005;3(3):249–58.
[8] Mircica E, Clutton RE, Kyles KW, et al. Problems associated with perioperative morphine in horses: a retrospective case analysis. Vet Anaesth Analg 2003;30(3):147–55.
[9] Thomasy SM, Slovis N, Maxwell LK, et al. Transdermal fentanyl combined with nonsteroidal anti-inflammatory drugs for analgesia in horses. J Vet Intern Med 2004;18(4):550–4.
[10] Aspenberg P. Drugs and fracture repair. Acta Orthop 2005;76(6):741–8.
[11] Lunn DP, Horohov DW. Immunomodulators. In: Reed SM, Bayly WM, Sellon DC, editors. Equine internal medicine. 2nd edition. St. Louis (MO): Saunders; 2006. p. 52–8.
[12] Slater MR, Hood DM, Carter GK. Descriptive epidemiological study of equine laminitis. International Journal of Applied Research in Veterinary Medicine 1995;27(5):364–7.
[13] Shuster R, Traub-Dargatz J, Baxter G. Survey of diplomates of the American College of Veterinary Internal Medicine and the American College of Veterinary Surgeons regarding clinical aspects and treatment of endotoxemia in horses. J Am Vet Med Assoc 1997;210(1):87–92.
[14] MacKay RJ. Brain injury after head trauma: pathophysiology, diagnosis, and treatment. Vet Clin North Am Equine Pract 2004;20(1):199–216.
[15] Day TK. Shock: pathophysiology, diagnosis, and treatment. In: Slatter D, editor. Textbook of small animal surgery. 3rd edition. Philadelphia: Saunders; 2003. p. 1–17.

[16] Bickell WH, Wall MJ, Pepe PE, et al. Immediate versus delayed fluid resuscitation for hypotensive patients with penetrating torso injuries. N Engl J Med 1994;331(17):1105–9.
[17] Cakir O, Subasi M, Erdem K, et al. Treatment of vascular injuries associated with limb fractures. Ann R Coll Surg Engl 2005;87:348–52.
[18] Cambridge H, Lees P, Hooke RE, et al. Antithrombotic actions of aspirin in the horse. Equine Vet J 1991;23(2):123–7.
[19] Broome TA, Brown MP, Gronwall RR, et al. Pharmacokinetics and plasma concentrations of acetylsalicylic acid after intravenous, rectal, and intragastric administration to horses. Can J Vet Res 2003;67(4):297–302.
[20] Feige K, Schwarzwald CC, Bombeli T. Comparison of unfractionated heparin and low molecular weight heparin for prophylaxis of coagulopathies in 52 horses with colic: a randomized double-blind clinical trial. Equine Vet J 2003;35(5):506–13.
[21] Moore BR, Hinchcliff KW. Heparin: a review of its pharmacology and therapeutic use in horses. J Vet Intern Med 1994;8(1):26–35.
[22] Martin GS. Factors associated with racing performance of Thoroughbreds undergoing lag screw repair of condylar fractures of the third metacarpal or third metatarsal bone. J Am Vet Med Assoc 2000;217(12):1870–7.
[23] Zekas LJ, Bramlage LR, Embertson RM, et al. Results of treatment of 145 fractures of the third metacarpal/metatarsal condyles in 135 horses (1986-1994). Equine Vet J 1999;31(4): 309–13.
[24] Carter BG, Schneider RK, Hardy J, et al. Assessment and treatment of equine humeral fractures: retrospective study of 54 cases (1972-1990). Equine Vet J 1993;25(3):203–7.
[25] Sweeney CR, Hodge TG. Sudden death in a horse following fracture of the acetabulum and iliac artery laceration. J Am Vet Med Assoc 1983;182(7):712–3.
[26] Rose PL, Watkins JP, Auer JA. Femoral fracture repair complicated by vascular injury in a foal. J Am Vet Med Assoc 1984;185(7):795–7.
[27] Rutkowski JA, Richardson DW. A retrospective study of 100 pelvic fractures in horses. Equine Vet J 1989;21(4):256–9.
[28] Little C, Hilbert B. Pelvic fractures in horses: 19 cases (1974-1984). J Am Vet Med Assoc 1987;190(9):1203–6.
[29] Richardson DW. Femur and pelvis. In: Auer JA, Stick JA, editors. Equine surgery. 3rd edition. St. Louis (MO): Saunders; 2006. p. 1334–41.
[30] Auer JA. Craniomaxillofacial disorders. In: Auer JA, Stick JA, editors. Equine surgery. 3rd edition. St. Louis (MO): Saunders; 2006. p. 1341–62.
[31] Henninger RW, Beard WL, Schneider RK, et al. Fractures of the rostral portion of the mandible and maxilla in horses: 89 cases (1979-1997). J Am Vet Med Assoc 1999;214(11): 1648–52.

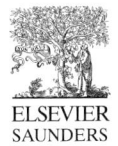

Oxidative Stress
Carl Soffler, DVM

Equine Internal Medicine, Department of Clinical Sciences, Colorado State University, College of Veterinary and Biomedical Sciences, 300 West Drake Road, Fort Collins, CO 80523, USA

Oxidative stress is most simply defined as an imbalance between oxidants and antioxidants in which the oxidant activity exceeds the neutralizing capability of antioxidants, resulting in cellular injury and activation of pathologic pathways [1,2]. Within this context, the oxidants of interest are collectively referred to as reactive oxygen species (ROS), which can be defined as oxygen-containing molecules that are more reactive than the triplet oxygen molecules present in air [2]. The biologically relevant molecules meeting this criterion include the superoxide anion radical, perhydroxyl radical, hydroxyl radical, and hydrogen peroxide. Additionally, nitric oxide (NO), nitrous anhydride, nitrogen dioxide, nitroxyl anion, peroxynitrite, and nitrosoperoxycarbonate can all be considered ROS but are more commonly referred to as reactive nitrogen species (RNS) [3,4].

The body is well equipped to deal with the production of these ROS with endogenous antioxidant scavenging systems, which include antioxidant enzymes, such as superoxide dismutase (SOD), catalase, and glutathione peroxidase (GPx). Additionally, there are numerous nonenzymatic antioxidants, which include α-tocopherol, β-carotene, ascorbic acid, ceruloplasmin, transferrin, albumin, glutathione, and uric acid among others [2,5]. When these systems are overwhelmed, as in the case of disease or extremes of physiologic stress, oxidant injury occurs.

Oxidative stress is an active field of research in human medicine and has been implicated in numerous disease processes ranging from sepsis to Alzheimer's disease [6]. ROS play active roles in the physiologic functions of proinflammatory signal transduction pathways, proliferation, programmed cell death, and inflammatory defense mechanisms (respiratory burst), in addition to causing cellular and tissue pathologic change through oxidation or free radical attack of cellular macromolecules [2,5,7]. Much attention has been focused on oxidant injury in human critical care patients and on its

E-mail address: csoffler@colostate.edu

role in the progression of critical illness through the systemic inflammatory response syndrome and multiorgan dysfunction. There is an established base of evidence for the importance of oxidative stress in critical illness in adults [5,8]. The natural progression of research in human critical care has been on the use of antioxidant therapies in an attempt to reduce morbidity and mortality. The results of such studies have been mixed, however, with only a few antioxidants proving to be efficacious to date [7,8].

A limited number of conditions in equine medicine have been investigated in regard to the effects of oxidative stress. In the field of critical care, this has been primarily limited to ischemia-reperfusion injury of the gastrointestinal tract. Recurrent airway obstruction (RAO) and exercise are two areas that have had some of the most research publications focusing on oxidative stress. Additionally, the role of oxidative stress has been described to varying degrees in osteoarthritis (OA), equine motor neuron disease (EMND), pituitary pars intermedia dysfunction (PPID), and endometritis. Studies in naturally affected horses as well as in experimental models have been used to evaluate the role of oxidant injury in disease as well as possible antioxidant therapies. As a relatively young field of research, there are numerous and rapidly evolving methodologies for evaluating oxidative stress, each with their own distinct advantages and disadvantages. Slight differences in models and methodologies make it difficult to make meaningful comparisons, even for studies that seem quite similar superficially. With this in mind, it is the goal of this review to summarize the present knowledge of oxidative stress in equine medicine and to examine the basis of and evidence for antioxidant therapy, highlighting the need for continued research on oxidative stress in equine medicine.

Conditions associated with oxidative stress

Ischemia-reperfusion injury

Oxidative stress is believed to be the underlying mechanism of reperfusion injury, which can be defined as continued tissue damage after the correction of ischemia and the return of blood flow. Ischemic injury is a distinct entity characterized by a critical reduction in blood flow and subsequent reduction in oxygen delivery [9]. It exists as a continuum, which depends on the severity and duration of the ischemia, ranging from mild cellular dysfunction to cell necrosis. Oxygen depletion causes a significant reduction of ATP production as glucose metabolism shifts from oxidative phosphorylation to anaerobic glycolysis. The resultant acidification of the intracellular environment causes denaturation of enzymes, which further inhibits ATP production [9]. Membrane ion pumps begin to fail as energy stores are further depleted, resulting in cellular swelling and further membrane dysfunction. This progresses to an influx of calcium ions, activation of phopholipase-A_2, degradation of membrane phospholipids, lysosomal enzyme release, autolysis, and irreversible cell necrosis or apoptosis [9].

Reperfusion injury depends on biochemical changes that occur during ischemia. The depletion of ATP during ischemia leads to an accumulation of AMP, which is further degraded to inosine and then to hypoxanthine [10]. Xanthine dehydrogenase (XDH) is converted to xanthine oxidase (XO) during the ischemic period by the calcium-dependent protease calpain [9,11]. When tissues are reperfused, XO catalyzes the oxidation of hypoxanthine to xanthine and uric acid, using oxygen as a cofactor and generating a superoxide radical [9,10]. The superoxide radical can cause damage by directly acting on biologic targets, but more effects seem to be from secondary formation of oxygen radicals. Superoxide undergoes a spontaneous second-order dismutation reaction yielding hydrogen peroxide and oxygen [3]. Hydrogen peroxide can then react with ferrous iron in the iron-catalyzed Fenton reaction to form the highly reactive hydroxyl radical. It was previously thought that the hydroxyl radical was produced by the Haber-Weiss reaction, but this has been shown to be incorrect when examined under physiologic conditions [3]. Superoxide also reacts with NO, forming peroxynitrite, another extremely reactive molecule [3]. These ROS cause direct damage to lipids, nucleic acids, and proteins and can initiate lipid peroxidation of organelle and cell membranes. In addition to causing direct damage, ROS indirectly stimulate neutrophil recruitment and activation through the generation of cytokines, particularly leukotriene B_4 and platelet-activating factor [9]. Neutrophils are the other half of the equation of reperfusion injury, providing another major source of ROS in reperfusion injury. Neutrophil myeloperoxidase (MPO) generates hypochlorous acid from hydrogen peroxide and chloride ions as part of the "respiratory burst" of activated neutrophils. They are thought to mediate much of the mucosal and microvascular injury, potentiating protein leakage and thrombus formation [9,10]. Neutrophils causing damage resulting in mucosal permeability seem to be primarily from the intestinal interstitium, whereas circulating leukocytes seem to mediate increases in microvascular permeability [10,12,13].

The actual role of reperfusion injury in the gastrointestinal tract of the horse is not quite as clear-cut as the previous summary of the pathophysiology, which has been described primarily from studies in rats, cats, and dogs. Many studies of ischemia-reperfusion injury in the horse have been conducted, with varied and conflicting results. Some of the discrepancies may result from the use of different models of ischemia-reperfusion injury (eg, low flow, partial or complete arterial, venous, arteriovenous ischemia) [13]. The small intestine and large colon seem to behave quite differently in response to ischemia reperfusion and should be considered separately in regard to this condition [14]. Furthermore, there is considerable debate and evidence to support the possibility that reperfusion injury may not be clinically relevant in the horse [12].

The small intestine of the horse seems to follow the previously described pathophysiology of ischemia and reperfusion described from other species. It has been demonstrated that XDH and XO are present in the small intestine of the horse, with a threefold increase in combined activity from the ileum to the duodenum. The percentage of XO activity does not vary significantly between segments, however. The percentage of XO activity did increase significantly after ischemic strangulation of 1 and 2 hours' duration [11]. This supports the possible role of XO in mediating oxygen free radical generation after ischemia. The basal levels and increase seen in XO are comparable to those seen in other species known to exhibit reperfusion injury [11,13]. Another study using a low-flow model of jejunal ischemia for 120 minutes followed by 120 minute of reperfusion failed to demonstrate any changes in XO activity, although increases in the severity of histologic lesions were seen during reperfusion [15]. However, it cannot be determined if the increase in lesion severity was continued injury from ischemia or separate reperfusion injury. Typically, low-flow models have produced the most compelling evidence for reperfusion injury [12,14,16]. These models have been used to evaluate different antioxidant therapies in reperfusion injury and are examined further during the consideration of specific antioxidants.

A model using venous strangulating obstruction (VSO; venous occlusion with continued arterial flow) of 90 minutes' duration followed by 90 minutes of reperfusion or another 90 minutes of ischemia showed no significant difference with or without reperfusion of lipid peroxidation or neutrophil infiltration [16]. VSO is a model considered to be the most consistent with naturally acquired lesions. After 90 minutes, there was a significant increase in lipid peroxidation, as measured by malondialdehyde levels, and neutrophil infiltration, as measured by tissue MPO [16]. This demonstrated the importance of ischemic injury to the jejunum with VSO to cause morphologic and biochemical changes but highlighted the fact that the damage caused by the ischemia is so great that any further injury caused by reperfusion is insignificant [16].

In addition to the role of XDH or XO and neutrophils in the pathogenesis of reperfusion injury, NO formed by inducible nitric oxide synthase (NOS) can be produced in excess and react with the superoxide anion to form peroxynitrite, resulting in lipid peroxidation and tissue damage [17]. Normally, endothelial NOS is protective to the mucosal barrier function, affecting vasodilation and decreasing neutrophil adhesion. During ischemia, it is thought that endothelial NOS is exhausted, eliminating its protective effects and resulting in the mucosal necrosis seen in ischemia-reperfusion injury [17]. In naturally occurring small intestinal strangulating obstruction, inducible NOS was found to localize to macrophages and eosinophils in the mucosa and submucosa, along with nitrotyrosine, which is another well-established marker of oxidant injury formed through the reactions of peroxynitrite [17]. Neutrophils are typically the leukocyte implicated in ischemia-reperfusion injury, and the fact that horses have a low number of neutrophils present in the interstitium has been one of the arguments against the occurrence of reperfusion injury in the horse [12,13,17,18]. The role of eosinophils and macrophages in ischemia or ischemia and reperfusion is currently unknown; however, they may play some of the roles in the horse that neutrophils have been shown to play in ischemia and reperfusion in laboratory animals [13,17].

Ischemia and reperfusion of the large colon as a naturally occurring condition is essentially limited to surgically corrected volvulus. The classic model of ischemia-reperfusion injury, which depends on XO, fails in the large colon, because the enzyme has only been detected at extremely low levels [9,12,14,19]. Despite numerous studies, convincing evidence of oxidative-based reperfusion injury is lacking [19–25]. One study found no evidence for oxidative stress during ischemia or reperfusion [14]. However, most studies have found evidence of some degree of oxidant injury. Ultrastructural and histologic reperfusion injury, as evidenced by rapid mucosal injury, has been demonstrated in the large colon in a low-flow model and in experimentally created torsions [24,25]. It has also been hypothesized that the reperfusion injury seen in the colon is a result of continued hypoxia, even after resolution of the volvulus, because of prolonged hypoperfusion (no reflow) [19]. Other studies have found evidence of oxidant injury (increased malondialdehyde [MDA] and decreased antioxidant defenses) associated with the ischemic phase, even though there was no evidence of reperfusion injury [22]. Elevated levels of MPO have also been found, indicating increased neutrophil infiltration as another source of oxidants [23]. Increased levels of inducible NOS and nitrotyrosine have only been demonstrated in mucosal leukocytes in horses with naturally acquired large colon volvulus. As in the small intestine, the predominant leukocytes found were eosinophils and macrophages. Increased levels of nitrotyrosine associated with peroxynitrite and mucosal damage were not seen during ischemia or reperfusion. This may be because of an inadequate period for NO formation, lack of superoxide production, or relatively small numbers of neutrophils [21].

The preponderance of conflicting studies of intestinal ischemia-reperfusion injury is nearly overwhelming. Most of the evidence supports a role of oxidative stress during some phase of ischemia or reperfusion. Some of the best studies illustrating reperfusion injury are low-flow models; however, these are generally not clinically relevant, except in cases of shock or prolonged distention [12,14]. Clinical patients typically have such severe ischemic injuries that any possible additional injury as a result of reperfusion is insignificant [12]. This should be kept in mind when considering the use of antioxidant therapies intended to treat ischemia-reperfusion injury, which is addressed later in this review.

Airway disease

In the horse, airway disease is often a key performance-limiting factor requiring lifelong therapy. ROS have been implicated in several human respiratory diseases, including adult respiratory distress syndrome, allergic asthma, chronic obstructive lung disease, and ozone exposure [6,26]. Research on equine airway disease and the role of oxidative stress has been primarily restricted to RAO. A role for oxidative stress has been hypothesized for exercise-induced pulmonary hemorrhage (EIPH), but no studies have demonstrated this relation to date [2,27].

One of the first studies of oxidant injury and the equine respiratory tract to determine the local and systemic effects of oxidative stress used a model of ozone exposure. Significant increases in reduced glutathione (GSH) and oxidized glutathione (GSSG) and in the glutathione redox ratio (GRR) [GRR = GSSG / (GSH + GSSG)] were seen in bronchoalveolar lavage fluid (BALF) after ozone exposure, which correlated well with endoscopic inflammatory scores. However, no changes were seen systemically in hemolysate values of GSH, GSSG, or the GRR [26]. Glutathione is one of the primary antioxidant defenses of the lungs and is present in the pulmonary epithelial lining fluid (PELF) in concentrations 100 times more than other extracellular tissue fluids [28].

A study comparing glutathione in the PELF and hemolysate of normal horses, horses with acute RAO disease, and horses with RAO in remission at rest demonstrated a clear role for oxidative stress in RAO. Compared with healthy horses, horses with RAO in crisis have elevated PELF GSH, GSSG, and GRR. How high levels of GSH are still maintained with increasing GSSG is unclear but is likely related to the unique ability of the lungs to maintain such high concentrations of GSH in PELF [28]. In cases of remission versus crisis in RAO, GSSG and the GRR are significantly higher, whereas GSH is unchanged. Again, the pathophysiologic mechanism for this is unknown but may be a result of endogenous oxidants from neutrophils, because the percentage of neutrophils in BALF correlates with BALF, GSSG, and GRR. The oxidative stress seen under these circumstances supports oxidant injury as an effect of airway inflammation and neutrophil activation rather than as a primary cause of pathologic change. The comparison of healthy horses with horses with RAO in remission revealed no statistical differences in PELF glutathione levels, even though an intermediate level of oxidative stress resulting from subclinical disease was suspected. As in the ozone model, no significant difference among any of the groups could be detected in markers of systemic oxidative stress [28].

Several similar studies were conducted comparing markers of oxidative stress in RAO-affected horses in response to exercise [29–31]. In one study, isoprostanes were used as the marker of interest to assess oxidant injury. Isoprostanes were significantly elevated in PELF and plasma after strenuous exercise in horses with RAO in remission compared with levels at rest. Horses with RAO in crisis had no significant difference in plasma isoprostanes but did have significantly higher PELF isoprostanes compared with horses with RAO in remission. Exercise in horses with an RAO crisis did increase plasma isoprostanes but did not cause significant change in PELF isoprostanes, which is not currently understood [29]. In pulmonary pathophysiology, 8-epi-prostaglandin $F_{2\alpha}$ ($PGF_{2\alpha}$) (an isoprostane) has been shown to be a marker of lipid peroxidation and a biologically active molecule that affects bronchoconstriction in human and laboratory animal studies. In one equine study, $PGF_{2\alpha}$ was shown to be an accurate marker of oxidant injury but did not have significant bronchoconstrictive properties [32].

In another study comparing healthy horses with horses with RAO in acute crisis and remission, glutathione, uric acid, and isoprostanes in plasma and PELF were compared with pulmonary function and airway inflammation [30]. At rest, horses with RAO in crisis and in remission were found to have significant elevations of hemolysate glutathione, indicating increased systemic synthesis of the antioxidant in response to RAO. Changes in the GRR demonstrated that oxidation of GSH to GSSG occurred primarily after exercise. Glutathione seemed to be the best systemic marker for increased oxidative stress in horses with RAO at rest. Uric acid was found to be increased by exercise in crisis and remission. Uric acid is formed by the enzymatic transformation of hypoxanthine to uric acid by XO or XDH, generating superoxide radicals just as in the gastrointestinal tract. This is thought to be related to lower oxygenation of blood (lower PaO_2) and subsequent delivery of oxygen to muscle, creating an environment favoring anaerobic glycolysis, ATP loss, and uric acid formation. Resting levels of uric acid did not seem to be directly related to RAO and impaired lung function. They seemed most useful as a systemic marker of oxidative stress in horses with RAO during exercise. Plasma isoprostanes did increase significantly during exercise in healthy horses and decrease significantly in horses with RAO in crisis. The decrease in isoprostanes could not be explained but, along with the increase seen in healthy horses, demonstrated that plasma levels of isoprostanes are not related to pulmonary oxidative stress and are more likely related to exercise-induced oxidative stress [30]. Local markers of oxidative stress in PELF, GSSG and isoprostanes, were significantly increased in horses with RAO in crisis, at rest, and after exercise, but no significant difference was found between these markers in normal horses and horses with RAO in remission. They significantly correlated with lung dysfunction, particularly PELF isoprostanes, which were significantly correlated with all measures of lung dysfunction, airway inflammation, and systemic glutathione status. There was no correlation between PELF and plasma isoprostanes [30].

Exercise intolerance is a frequent complaint of horses with RAO. A study comparing exercise tolerance in six RAO horses while in crisis and remission (two separate time points) showed a significant reduction during crisis but no significant difference in markers of oxidative stress in horses in crisis. Horses in remission did have significant increases in the GRR and plasma lipid hydroperoxides (LPHs) after exercise. At rest, horses in crisis had significantly higher maximal pleural pressures and total pulmonary resistance and significantly lower dynamic compliance and PaO_2 than horses in remission, which is consistent with bronchoconstriction and impaired oxygenation [33]. The hypoxemia observed at rest remained consistently higher at maximal exercise and after exercise. The lack of oxidative stress in horses with RAO in crisis and its presence in horses with RAO with remission during exercise were hypothesized to be a result of the intensity and duration of exercise achieved or the level of hypoxemia present during exercise [33]. The mechanism and role of oxidative stress in exercise are examined further in the next section.

One study has been conducted specifically evaluating summer pasture–associated obstructive pulmonary disease (SPAOPD). No significant differences were found in plasma or BALF NO concentrations, percentage of bronchial epithelial cells staining positive for nicotinamide adenine dinucleotide phosphate diaphorase (NADPHd) or nitrotyrosine, or leukocyte staining positive for NADPHd, nitrotyrosine, or inducible NOS when comparing normal and SPAOPD-affected horses. The only significant difference was in the percentage of bronchial epithelial cells staining positive for inducible NOS. The authors concluded that NO is probably not a major mediator of airway inflammation but that it could play a role in the amplification of an inflammatory airway response. Furthermore, the lack of nitrotyrosine staining indicates a lack of superoxide production. If superoxide was present, some degree of nitrotyrosine staining would be expected because it would react with the NO known to be present [34]. This does not support a role for oxidative stress in SPAOPD; however, other markers of pulmonary oxidant injury, such as the PELF GRR and isoprostanes, were not assessed.

Exercise

Studies in human beings and laboratory animals have demonstrated that strenuous and prolonged low- to medium-intensity exercise induces oxidative stress [35–37]. The widespread use of horses as athletes has generated much interest in the role of oxidant injury during exercise in terms of the physiology of muscle fatigue, pathophysiology of myopathies, increasing performance with antioxidants, and welfare issues. The formation of ROS during exercise is caused primarily by the increase in mitochondrial respiration associated with the increased energy demands made during exercise [36,38,39]. There may also be increased ROS from activated phagocytes and enzymes (oxidases). These are physiologic processes that overwhelm the endogenous antioxidant defenses because of the intensity or duration of exercise [38]. Skeletal muscle may be a primary site of oxidant injury because it seems to have comparatively low levels of antioxidants [39].

Higher levels of oxygen consumption during exercise have also been implicated as a factor contributing to oxidative stress in human beings [36]. At rest, 1% to 5% of oxygen is incompletely reduced and forms ROS, such as superoxide [36,40,41]. In human beings, strenuous exercise has been shown to increase oxygen uptake up to 200 times that of resting levels [40]. An elite human athlete consumes oxygen at a rate of 70 mL/kg^{-1}/min^{-1}, whereas a horse can consume oxygen at a rate as high as 200 mL/kg^{-1}/min^{-1}. This suggests that the horse has the potential for significant oxidative stress during exercise and should have well-developed antioxidant defenses to deal with these high levels of oxygen metabolism [36]. Several studies have been conducted to evaluate the effects of different types of exercise. There are certainly discrepancies among the studies, but there are also significant differences in study design and markers of oxidative stress measured [2]. Several studies have also used oxidative stress during exercise as a method to evaluate different antioxidant therapies; these findings are examined during the discussion of individual antioxidant therapies.

Endurance racing is a good model of prolonged medium-intensity exercise that would be expected to produce oxidative stress. One study compared horses in two 80-km races similar in terrain but different in ambient temperature (5.5°C versus 28°C). The race conducted at a higher ambient temperature had significant postrace decreases in vitamin C, GSH, and GPx and significantly higher levels of creatine kinase (CK) and aspartate aminotransferase (AST). These changes were evident immediately after the race and after a 1-hour recovery period. The race at a lower ambient temperature only showed a significant decrease in GSH [42]. These findings were consistent with those of an earlier study that found significant differences in oxidative stress in horses exercised at high and low levels of heat stress [43]. Vitamin E concentrations were unchanged throughout and after exercise. The authors hypothesized that vitamin E was maintained at the expense of vitamin C and GSH and that the increases in CK and AST were a result of oxidative stress causing muscle cell damage and leakage [42]. A similar study using a 140-km race also showed significant reductions in total glutathione (TGSH) and increased total barbituric acid reactive substances (TBARs), CK, and AST immediately after the race. Significant reductions in vitamin C and the GRR were seen after 16 hours of recovery. The vitamin E levels were unchanged by racing in this study as well [35].

Another study using racehorses found evidence of oxidative stress but not muscle damage after a standardized exercise protocol. The horses were trained for 3 months and then challenged with a short-duration high-intensity exercise test. Controlled training is one proposed method to increase the endogenous antioxidant defenses to protect against exercise-induced oxidative stress [44]. Despite the training program, the horses still had elevated levels of MDA immediately and 18 hours after exercise. GSH levels peaked immediately after exercise, demonstrating the induction of antioxidant defenses, and there was no evidence of muscle injury as a result of oxidative stress, with no statistically significant increases in CK or lactate dehydrogenase isoenzyme 4 (LDH-4) [44]. Whether the lack of muscle enzyme elevation was attributable to the training or to the design of the exercise test cannot be determined.

A study of Standardbred trotters was conducted specifically to evaluate the antioxidant capacity of the horses after induction by a single bout of moderate exercise and its ability to prevent oxidative stress, as measured by LPHs [36]. The trotters were all regularly trained to treadmill exercise before a 53-minute session of moderate intensity. The antioxidant capacity was assessed by oxygen radical absorbance capacity (ORAC). After exercise, there was a significant increase in ORAC, which remained increased through a 24-hour recovery period. Despite this increase, LPHs were significantly increased after exercise, indicating that the physiologic increase in antioxidant protection was not great enough to prevent lipid peroxidation. There were no significant changes in vitamin E or TGSH. The study did suggest that increased pre-exercise antioxidant capacity might be able to limit the extent of exercise-induced oxidative stress [36].

Equine motor neuron disease

EMND is a neurodegenerative disease of the somatic lower motor neuron system of the adult horse [2,45]. Histopathologic evidence of oxidative stress is seen by the predominance of type I muscle fiber atrophy and lipopigment deposition in the capillaries of the spinal cord and retinal pigment epithelium [45,46]. Type I fibers are hypothesized to be preferentially affected because of the greater oxidative activity of the parent motor neurons [46]. Vitamin E deficiency, which is associated with lack of access to fresh pasture, is a risk factor for EMND [45]. However, vitamin E deficiency is not the sole cause of EMND, as evidenced by attempts to create the disease experimentally and by findings in naturally occurring cases. Vitamin E may be low because of its consumption during antioxidant defenses as well as a deficiency in dietary antioxidants [46]. Additionally, elevated levels of copper (Cu) have been found in the spinal cords of horses affected with EMND. There are two hypotheses to explain the significance of the increased Cu concentrations. The Cu could accumulate from increased concentrations of Cu-zinc (Zn) SOD, which would be a reflection of free radical activity in the spinal cord [47]. The similarities between EMND and amyotrophic lateral sclerosis (ALS; Lou Gehrig's disease), for which there is a known defect in Cu-Zn SOD, has led to the investigation of the equine gene for Cu-Zn SOD in horses affected with EMND. To date, no comparable mutations in the gene for equine Cu-Zn SOD have been found, and there is no evidence to support a link between EMND and any mutations of Cu-Zn SOD [48]. Accumulation of Cu may occur for another pathophysiologic reason but ultimately induces free radical formation by means of the Fenton reaction, as would iron, forming hydroxyl ions [45,47]. Additionally, extremely high levels of hepatic Cu have been found in horses with experimentally induced EMND but not in naturally occurring disease [47]. High levels of hepatic and serum iron also have been found in horses with naturally occurring EMND but not in experimental animals, although there are not elevated levels of spinal cord iron in horses affected by EMND. If total body antioxidant defenses are depleted (including vitamin E), these horses should be more susceptible to oxidative stress if there are elevations in iron [45]. The cumulative effects of the antioxidant and pro-oxidant burden, regardless of its origin, seem to be critical in EMND, but there is still much to be learned about the pathogenesis of this disease.

Joint disease

OA is an active area of equine research because it is a common cause of poor performance and early retirement [49]. However, little research has been conducted on the role of oxidative stress in OA in human beings or horses compared with the total body of research conducted on OA. One of the earlier studies used a carrageenin model of synovitis but was unable to document a significant difference between carrageenin- and saline-injected controls. This study was limited in that it was conducted before the development of many quantitative assays for oxidative stress. The study did suggest that increased numbers of activated phagocytic cells attracted to joints inflamed with carrageenin produced superoxide during the respiratory burst, leading to free radical production [50].

Another study examining the role of ROS in equine joint disease evaluated the difference in the protein carbonyl content of synovial fluid as a marker of oxidative stress in acute joint disease compared with that in normal joints. Horses had joints affected by traumatic injury (primarily chip fragmentation) or osteochondritis dissecans (OCD). In either case, the protein carbonyl content was significantly higher than in control horses [51]. ROS have been proposed to cause damage by decreasing the viscosity of hyaluronan by breaking it into smaller chains. This decreases viscosity, increases friction, and eliminates the ability of hyaluronan to inhibit phagocytosis by polymorphonuclear leukocytes, which, when activated, produce more free radicals as part of the respiratory burst. The ROS can cause direct damage to collagen, decrease proteoglycan synthesis, impair chondrocyte energy metabolism, and cause cell death. The primary antioxidants of the equine joint to protect from this oxidant injury are thought to be ceruloplasmin and transferrin [51]. A trend toward a significant increase in the antioxidant status of the affected joints was found, which was not expected but matches the induction of antioxidant defenses seen in exercise models of oxidative stress [36,51]. However, the increased antioxidant status may have been affected by the use of phenylbutazone to treat pain and swelling associated with the injury or surgical procedure [51].

Most recently, two studies have investigated the presence of nitrotyrosine in equine cartilage and bone in joints affected by OA [49,52]. One study focused on chondrocyte apoptosis because it has been implicated as a major pathway of OA development. The study found a significantly higher percentage of apoptotic chondrocytes in degenerative articular cartilage, with the areas of apoptotic chondrocytes colocalizing with positive nitrotyrosine staining. This suggests a close interrelation of oxidative stress, chondrocyte apoptosis, and cartilage matrix degeneration, but the precise nature of this relation is unknown [49]. Another study found that nitrotyrosine staining was significantly elevated in the subchondral bone of horses with OA compared with controls, although not in cartilage or trabecular bone layers, indicating a role of oxidative stress in this layer in the development of early or moderate OA [52].

Equine pituitary pars intermedia dysfunction (equine Cushing's disease)

Equine PPID is one of the most common diseases of aged ponies and horses. Despite recognition as a clinical entity for more than 70 years, its pathophysiology is relatively poorly understood [53]. Recently, oxidative stress has been implicated in equine PPID, partially because of some similarities to human diabetics. Horses with PPID are often insulin resistant, with abnormal glucose and insulin levels. Oxidative stress secondary to hyperglycemia has been clearly associated with microvascular dysfunction in human diabetics and was proposed as a possible contributing factor for laminitis, which is often seen in horses and ponies with PPID [54]. However, there is little evidence to support systemic oxidative stress in PPID. The only systemic marker of oxidative stress found to be significantly different in horses with PPID compared with control horses is plasma thiols, but even these are not significant if corrected for albumin concentration [54]. Plasma MDA and nitrotyrosine, as measures of systemic oxidative stress, as well as red blood cell GPx, SOD, and GSH, as measures of systemic antioxidant capacity, showed no significant difference in controls and horses with PPID [54,55].

There is evidence to support local oxidative stress within the pars intermedia. Positive nitrotyrosine staining of the pars intermedia was significantly greater in horses with PPID compared with age-matched controls. There was also a similar decrease in the tyrosine hydroxylase–staining cells in horses with PPID, supporting the loss of functional dopaminergic neurons in the pathophysiology of PPID. Additionally, the staining seen in the aged controls versus the young controls was significantly greater, demonstrating an age-related accumulation of a marker of oxidative stress [53]. In regard to the antioxidant capacity of the pars intermedia, GPx activity was found to increase, along with nitrotyrosine. No correlations between TGSH, total SOD, or magnesium (Mg)-SOD and oxidative stress were found. There was a significant age-associated decrease in Mg-SOD but no significant correlation between TGSH, total SOD, or GPx and age [55]. Thus, there does not seem to be a significant decrease in the antioxidant capacity of the pars intermedia in equine Cushing's disease. Even though there is an age-associated decrease in Mg-SOD, there is no correlation between nitrotyrosine and Mg-SOD. However, the lack of increase in Mg-SOD with aging could be interpreted as a failure of induction of appropriate antioxidant defenses, and could thus represent a functional deficiency that increases the risk of PPID in older horses [55].

Other conditions associated with oxidative stress

Additional disease associations with oxidative stress have been described in the literature on a more limited basis. Acute colitis, naturally occurring and induced in a castor oil model of colitis, has been shown to be associated with increased MDA and MPO, predominantly of eosinophilic origin, which correlated with the severity of histologic tissue damage [56,57]. Endometritis has been shown to be associated with significantly increased levels of plasma MDA and decreased red blood cell GPx activity in Arabian mares [58]. A series of horses examined for severe cutaneous burns were also seen to have evidence of oxidative stress, detectable as morphologic changes in erythrocytes (eccentrocytes, spherocytoid cells, formation of Heinz-body-like structures, and membrane blebbing with fragmentation) as a result of cell membrane damage [59]. There is still much to learn about many of the disease processes in equine medicine. Nevertheless, it seems quite certain that oxidative stress is going to be found to play an important role in more and more conditions as the underlying pathophysiology is discovered.

Therapeutic antioxidants

Despite the well-established role of oxidant injury in human medicine and the association with poor outcomes in critically ill patients, the evidentiary basis for therapeutic antioxidant supplementation is weak. Supplementation has been shown to improve antioxidant capacity, but whether this actually produces a clinical benefit is still uncertain. A recent meta-analysis found that parenteral selenium was the only supplement associated with a reduction in mortality in acute intensive care unit conditions [7]. Similarly, the importance of antioxidant deficiencies in exercise-induced oxidative stress and exercise intolerance is well known, whereas the benefit of antioxidant supplementation on performance is not, although antioxidant supplementation is widely practiced in human athletes [38]. In equine medicine, the effects of antioxidant therapy have been evaluated to varying degrees during exercise, reperfusion injury, RAO, and basal conditions. The following section summarizes the mechanism of action of antioxidants evaluated in the horse and their evidence of efficacy in treating oxidative stress.

Vitamin E and selenium

Vitamin E (α-tocopherol) resides in the lipophilic center of cell membranes. It is unique in that it is the only antioxidant capable of breaking the chain reaction of lipid peroxidation. When vitamin E is transformed into its radical state, it is weakly reactive and thus prevents further oxidation of adjacent polyunsaturated fatty acids [1]. Experimentally, vitamin E is infrequently evaluated alone and is usually found in some combination with vitamin C or selenium. One study evaluated the effect of vitamin E status on lipid peroxidation during treadmill exercise. The model was not able to produce oxidative stress consistently. Plasma vitamin E did significantly negatively correlate with plasma TBARs ($r = -0.398$), but there were no significant effects on performance [60]. Another study comparing horses supplemented with vitamin E at a dose 300 mg/kg greater than National Research Council (NRC) levels and standard NRC levels, found no difference in erythrocyte SOD and catalase activity before, immediately after, or 30 minutes after strenuous treadmill running. The activity of GPx was significantly higher in horses supplemented with vitamin E 30 minutes after exercise. The authors concluded that additional dietary supplementation provided no benefit to antioxidant defense. However, no measures of oxidative stress were tested [37].

Selenium is a trace mineral required for the function of GPx. Although it is considered an essential nutrient, there is not a clearly defined syndrome of deficiency [1]. The effect of 70 days of training and supplementation of vitamin E and selenium on MDA, total peroxyl-radical trapping (TRAP), GPx activity and content, in vitro erythrocyte resistance to oxidative stress, and plasma vitamin E was evaluated with a standardized performance test in 11 3-year-old stallions in a repeated measures design [39]. Vitamin E was quite low before training and supplementation, and exercise produced no effect on plasma levels. After training and supplementation, it was significantly higher but still decreased throughout the second performance test. Before and after the 70-day period, the exercise test produced significant increases in MDA, although the increase was significantly less after training and supplementation. Vitamin E content and MDA were significantly inversely correlated throughout the experiment. Erythrocyte resistance to oxidative stress and TRAP were significantly increased by the protocol. No statistical difference in GPx content or activity could be shown [39]. This study demonstrated a clear enhancement of antioxidant capacity and reduction in oxidative stress as a result of training and supplementation with vitamin E and selenium. However, without additional control groups, it is not possible to determine which, if any, of each of these treatments was primarily responsible for the observed improvement.

Vitamin C

Vitamin C (ascorbic acid) is a water-soluble antioxidant, which acts through its ability to donate electrons (reducing agent) to ROS and is essential for the regeneration of vitamin E and other antioxidants from their oxidized forms [1,61]. Vitamin C can also have pro-oxidant effects in presence of iron and copper, resulting in the production of hydroxyl radicals [1]. The horse is unique in that it has the ability to synthesize vitamin C and does not depend on dietary intake [61,62]. Vitamin C is the most abundant nonenzymatic antioxidant in the lung and is concentrated in the PELF 100 times greater than plasma [62]. These high levels are 20 times the level in human beings and are thought to reflect the horse's ability to synthesize vitamin C [61]. The effectiveness and need for vitamin C supplementation were investigated in one paper, which found that oral supplementation with ascorbyl palmitate (AP) or calcium ascorbyl-2-monophosphate (CAP) could significantly increase BALF ascorbic acid concentrations, but only AP produced a significant increase in plasma vitamin C. No cytologic changes in tracheal wash or BALF samples were observed with 2 weeks of supplementation, nor were there any changes in BALF oxidant status (uric acid, GSH, and GSSG) other than vitamin C concentrations [62]. Horses affected with RAO have been shown to have reduced levels of plasma ascorbic acid compared with healthy animals. Horses with RAO with active airway inflammation have significantly lower concentrations of PELF ascorbic acid compared with horses without inflammation, which also have significantly lower PELF ascorbic acid concentrations compared with control horses. This suggests that there is local and systemic oxidative stress occurring in these horses as a result of decreased production, increased consumption, sequestration, or metabolism of vitamin C [61]. However, the clinical benefit of vitamin C supplementation in these horses has not been well evaluated.

Two studies have examined the use of vitamin C in reducing oxidative stress associated with exercise. No difference in any marker of antioxidant capacity or oxidative stress, other than plasma ascorbate levels, was found after 3 weeks of supplementation with vitamin E at a dose of 5000 IU with or without vitamin C at a dose of 7 g/d administered orally in a paired group of 23 endurance horses before, during, or after an 80-km race. Plasma ascorbate was significantly increased in the vitamin E and C groups. There was consistent evidence of oxidative stress and muscle leakage in both groups, indicating that there was no benefit to supplementation with vitamin C [41]. The value of vitamin E supplementation could not be assessed, because there was no control group for vitamin E. Intravenous supplementation of ascorbate at a dose of 5g immediately before racing in Thoroughbred racehorses prevented increased production of TBARs and maintained stable values for plasma antioxidant capacity (PAOC) and total antioxidant reactivity (TAR) after racing. Untreated animals had increased TBARs and reduced PAOC and TAR. All animals had increased muscle leakage enzymes. Thus, vitamin C seemed to be able to limit oxidative stress but could not prevent muscle membrane damage associated with high-intensity short-duration exercise [63].

Multiple vitamin or mineral supplementation

Supplementation with various combinations of vitamins and minerals has been evaluated in a handful of studies, primarily in terms of pulmonary function and disease. One study examined the effect of an antioxidant feed supplement containing vitamins C, E, and B as well as Cu, Zn, and selenium on plasma ascorbic acid and the PAOC of water and lipid-soluble components, vitamin E, vitamin B, selenium, Cu, Zn, whole-blood GSH and GSSG, SOD, and GPx in trained Thoroughbred racehorses during a 3-month training and racing period. Supplemented horses had significant increases in the PAOC of water and lipid-soluble components, vitamin E, vitamin B, selenium, and erythrocyte GPx activity. A significant increase in plasma CK seen in the control group was notably absent in the supplemented group. Significant increases in GSSG and the GRR and decreases in GSH were seen in both groups over the course of the study, with no difference demonstrated with supplementation [38]. The study did not evaluate any difference in performance between the two groups despite the apparent benefit of the supplement on the oxidant-antioxidant imbalance generated during racing and race training.

The effect of supplementation with vitamins E and C, along with selenium, has been evaluated in healthy horses and horses with RAO in remission. In healthy horses, the only significant changes seen after 4 weeks of supplementation, before and after a standard exercise test, were increased levels of plasma vitamins E and C. The authors concluded that additional antioxidant supplementation has no apparent benefit (or detriment) to pulmonary function during moderate exercise in healthy horses, assuming that their diet is not deficient in antioxidants. The exercise test did not induce oxidative stress in either group as measured by the PELF MDA, GRR, and ascorbic acid redox ratio [64]. A similar supplement and exercise test regimen in horses with RAO improved exercise tolerance, reduced gross visible airway inflammation, and decreased plasma uric acid, presumably from downregulation of the XDH-XO pathway. Supplementation did not affect the significant increases in plasma isoprostanes seen in both groups, nor did it significantly change any measures of oxidative stress in the PELF [65]. Another study with a similar design examining this supplementation in horses with RAO was not able to replicate the induction of systemic or pulmonary oxidative stress and only documented significant increases in plasma vitamins E and C as a result of supplementation [66].

N-acetylcysteine

N-acetylcysteine (NAC) is a glutathione analogue, which has been primarily utilized only for its mucolytic properties in the horse. It readily crosses cell membranes; replenishes depleted glutathione stores; scavenges ROS directly; increases cyclic guanosine monophosphate, causes vasodilation and inhibits platelet aggregation; and can reduce proinflammatory cytokine production [1,5]. In human medicine, it is the treatment of choice for acetaminophen toxicity and is under considerable investigation for the treatment of many other disease processes. In the horse, NAC has been examined as an antiprotease for the cornea and RAO-affected lungs. However, its use specifically as an antioxidant in the horse has only been investigated in an in vitro model of mucosal injury and restitution in the right dorsal colon. Pretreatment with NAC was found to prevent hypochlorous acid–induced tissue damage, changes in resistance, and eosinophil migration but did not prevent increased mannitol permeability [67].

Allopurinol

Allopurinol is a structural analogue of hypoxanthine, and thus acts as an XO inhibitor through competition with hypoxanthine in the XO-catalyzed conversion of hypoxanthine to uric acid. The benefits of allopurinol in ischemia-reperfusion injury have been seen after long-term oral administration, which has little practical application in the horse. There was no benefit observed with intravenous administration of allopurinol after experimental ischemia but before reperfusion of the small intestine or large colon of equids [9]. Intravenous and oral allopurinol supplementation has been shown to inhibit XO effectively during an exercise test, resulting in significantly higher hypoxanthine and xanthine levels and lower LPH, GSSG, and GRR levels in treated versus control horses [40]. Another study demonstrated that pretreatment with allopurinol intraperitoneally significantly reduced the rise in XO activity in response to intraperitoneally administered endotoxin but did not evaluate the efficacy of allopurinol as a treatment after the initiation of endotoxic shock [68].

Dimethyl sulfoxide

Dimethyl sulfoxide (DMSO) has anti-inflammatory and antioxidant properties and acts by scavenging hydroxyl radicals, inhibiting the production of interleukin-8 and subsequent neutrophil chemotaxis, stabilizing lysosomal membranes, inhibiting platelet aggregation, and inhibiting fibroblast proliferation [9,10]. Studies in cats and rats have shown that DMSO attenuates microvascular permeability and neutrophil infiltration associated with ischemia and reperfusion when used as a pretreatment [10]. Studies evaluating the efficacy of DMSO in the equine gastrointestinal tract have produced inconsistent results [9]. Experimentally, DMSO has not been shown to provide any benefit in ischemia-reperfusion injury of the large colon, and one study demonstrated increased mucosal damage in horses treated with DMSO [9,10,20]. The effect of DMSO in the small intestine has been more variable, with some studies showing no benefit (1 g/kg administered intravenously), whereas others have shown that DMSO (20 mg/kg administered intravenously) decreases microvascular permeability and limits cellular infiltrate but does cause mild submucosal and serosal edema [9,10]. A study in foals showed that DMSO (20 mg/kg administered intravenously) prevented small intestinal adhesion formation in foals after ischemia-reperfusion injury [69]. However, antioxidant capacity and oxidative stress were not measured in many of these studies, such that the possible benefits of DMSO cannot necessarily be attributed to its antioxidant action. It has been hypothesized that the dose necessary for hydroxyl radical scavenging may be toxic to cells [9].

21-Aminosteroids (U-74389G)

The 21-aminosteroids are derivatives of glucocorticoids. The modification eliminates the ability of the molecule to activate the corticosteroid receptor [9]. They scavenge superoxide radicals and lipid hydroperoxides, preventing iron-catalyzed lipid peroxidation and arachidonic acid release [10]. Their ability to limit lipid peroxidation has been shown to limit gastrointestinal ischemia-reperfusion injury and MDA concentration in dogs and laboratory animals [9,10]. Evaluation of U-74389G in ischemia and reperfusion of the large colon did not significantly alter tissue MDA or MPO concentrations, but the model used was not able to create significant increases in either of these variables in the control horses. U-74389G was able to prevent a reduction in mucosal surface area associated with ischemia [70]. A similar study of the small intestine using models of total and partial vascular occlusion found that U-74389G did not prevent a reduction in mucosal surface area. This study also failed to produce significant elevations in tissue MDA or MPO in its control horses, and there was no effect of U-74389G on these values either [71]. A more recent study found that U-74389G had no effect on microvascular permeability, increased submucosal and serosal edema, and caused moderate cellular infiltration. The authors concluded that there was not a benefit to treatment with U-74389G, and it may cause mucosal injury [10].

Carolina rinse

Carolina rinse (CR) is a solution that was developed as a perfusate to store donated organs before transplantation, with the goal of minimizing reperfusion injury. It is composed of allopurinol and glutathione (antioxidants), deferoxamine (iron chelator), nicardipine (calcium channel blocker), ATP substrates, fructose, glucose, adenosine, and modified hydroxyethyl starch with a solution pH of 6.5 [72]. It has been evaluated as a local treatment for ischemia-reperfusion injury of equine jejunum in low-flow models. Local treatment has consisted of topical, intraluminal, and intra-arterial perfusion of jejunal vessels, which has fairly consistently been reported to prevent increases in microvascular permeability, reduce neutrophil migration and edema, and decrease fibroplasia [10,72,73]. However, it was not protective to microvascular permeability in models using jejunal distention [73]. There was no appreciable subjective clinical benefit seen in the horses treated with CR [72]. This, in combination with the greatest apparent benefit achieved from intra-arterial perfusion, may account for the limited clinical use of CR.

A customized solution composed of glutamine, adenosine, allopurinol, deferoxamine, DMSO, prostaglandin E_1, and dextrose in a base of lactated Ringer's solution was evaluated for intra-arterial and intraluminal efficacy in preventing ischemia-reperfusion injury in an in vitro low-flow model of equine jejunum. The solution had significant protective effects in minimizing ischemia-reperfusion injury in terms of histomorphologic injury and mucosal permeability to albumin [74,75].

Future antioxidant therapies

Future research should undoubtedly continue to expand the current understanding of oxidative stress and provide new targets to treat. Novel antioxidants continue to be discovered; however, the greatest potential for future therapies seems to lie in the development of artificial enzymes ("synzymes"), which should enable breakthrough of the stoichiometric limitations of all the current antioxidant therapies [3]. Synthetic SOD and peroxynitrite decomposition catalysts have been developed [3,4]. A synthetic formulation of SOD has recently been developed and marketed for dogs (Oxstrin, Nutramx Laboratories, Edgewood, Maryland).

Manganese chloride, a simple inorganic salt, has been investigated in the horse for its ability to mimic the action of SOD. It is clearly less effective than SOD but seems safe and is considerably less expensive than SOD mimetics [10,76]. Furthermore, it is stable, making oral administration possible [76]. Only limited studies have been conducted with it, however, and it failed to reduce mucosal injury in a model of large colon ischemia-reperfusion injury [10].

Summary

The field of oxidative stress research and evidence-based antioxidant therapy in equine medicine is still in the early stages of development. There is a great deal to be discovered about the importance and basic pathophysiology of oxidative stress in horses. Even as oxidant injury is proven to be associated with numerous conditions, it still remains to be seen if it is a primary cause of pathologic change or a secondary effect of disease processes. The field of human medicine, which is far ahead in this area, is still struggling to prove the clinical benefit of antioxidant therapy [5,7]. The clinical use of antioxidants in human beings and animals alike is becoming increasingly common as there is more awareness of the importance of oxidative stress. The low cost and minimal side effects associated with antioxidants promote their use as well, despite a lack of evidence for their use. The hope is that future research can better demonstrate the clinical importance of oxidative stress and tangible benefits of specific antioxidant supplementation therapies.

References

[1] Marino PL. Oxidant injury. In: Wingfield WE, Raffe MR, editors. The veterinary ICU book. Jackson (WY): Teton Newmedia; 2002. p. 24–39.
[2] Kirschvink N, Lekeux P. Pferdeheilkunde. [Oxidative stress in equine medicine—current knowledge]. 2002;18(6):569–73 [in German].
[3] Cuzzocrea S, Riley DP, Caputi AP, et al. Antioxidant therapy: a new pharmacological approach in shock, inflammation, and ischemia/reperfusion injury. Pharmacol Rev 2001; 53(1):135–59.
[4] Olmos A, Giner RM, Manez S. Drugs modulating the biological effects of peroxynitrite and related nitrogen species. Med Res Rev 2006; [Jun 2, Epub ahead of print].
[5] Crimi E, Sica V, Williams-Ignarro S, et al. The role of oxidative stress in adult critical care. Free Radic Biol Med 2006;40(3):398–406.
[6] Fam SS, Morrow JD. The isoprostanes: unique products of arachidonic acid oxidation—a review. Curr Med Chem 2003;10(17):1723–40.
[7] Heyland DK, Dhaliwal R, Suchner U, et al. Antioxidant nutrients: a systematic review of trace elements and vitamins in the critically ill patient. Intensive Care Med 2005;31(3): 327–37.
[8] Nathens AB, Neff MJ, Jurkovich GJ, et al. Randomized, prospective trial of antioxidant supplementation in critically ill surgical patients. Ann Surg 2002;236(6):814–22.
[9] Moore RM, Muir WW, Granger DN. Mechanisms of gastrointestinal ischemia-reperfusion injury and potential therapeutic interventions: a review and its implications in the horse. J Vet Intern Med 1995;9(3):115–32.
[10] Dabareiner RM, White NA, Snyder JR, et al. Effects of Carolina rinse solution, dimethyl sulfoxide, and the 21-aminosteroid, U-74389G, on microvascular permeability and morphology of the equine jejunum after low-flow ischemia and reperfusion. Am J Vet Res 2005;66(3):525–36.
[11] Prichard M, Ducharme NG, Wilkins PA, et al. Xanthine oxidase formation during experimental ischemia of the equine small intestine. Can J Vet Res 1991;55(4):310–4.
[12] Blikslager AT, Roberts MC, Gerard MP, et al. How important is intestinal reperfusion injury in horses? J Am Vet Med Assoc 1997;211(11):1387–9.
[13] Moore RM. Clinical relevance of intestinal reperfusion injury in horses. J Am Vet Med Assoc 1997;211(11):1362–6.
[14] Kooreman K, Babbs C, Fessler J. Effect of ischemia and reperfusion on oxidative processes in the large colon and jejunum of horses. Am J Vet Res 1998;59(3):340–6.
[15] Vatistas NJ, Snyder JR, Nieto J, et al. Morphologic changes and xanthine oxidase activity in the equine jejunum during low flow ischemia and reperfusion. Am J Vet Res 1998;59(6):772–6.
[16] Laws EG, Freeman DE. Significance of reperfusion injury after venous strangulation obstruction of equine jejunum. J Invest Surg 1995;8(4):263–70.
[17] Mirza MH, Oliver JL, Seahorn TL, et al. Detection and comparison of nitric oxide in clinically normal horses and those with naturally acquired small intestinal strangulation obstruction. Can J Vet Res 1999;63(4):230–40.
[18] Gerard MP, Blikslager AT, Roberts MC, et al. The characteristics of intestinal injury peripheral to strangulating obstruction lesions in the equine small intestine. Equine Vet J 1999; 31(4):331–5.

[19] Wilkins PA, Ducharme NG, Lowe JE, et al. Measurements of blood flow and xanthine oxidase activity during postischemic reperfusion of the large colon of ponies. Am J Vet Res 1994;55(8):1168–77.
[20] Reeves MJ, Vansteenhouse J, Stashak TS, et al. Failure to demonstrate reperfusion injury following ischaemia of the equine large colon using dimethyl sulphoxide. Equine Vet J 1990;22(2):126–32.
[21] Mirza MH, Seahorn TL, Oliver JL, et al. Detection and comparison of nitric oxide in clinically healthy horses and those with naturally acquired strangulating large colon volvulus. Can J Vet Res 2005;69(2):106–15.
[22] Sullivan KE, Snyder JR, Schiedt MJ, et al. Lipid peroxidation and antioxidant defences during ischaemia and reperfusion of the equine ascending colon. Equine Vet J Suppl 1992;13: 99–101.
[23] Grulke S, Benbarek H, Caudron I, et al. Plasma myeloperoxidase level and polymorphonuclear leukocyte activation in horses suffering from large intestinal obstruction requiring surgery: preliminary results. Can J Vet Res 1999;63(2):142–7.
[24] Meschter CL, Craig D, Hackett R. Histopathological and ultrastructural changes in simulated large colonic torsion and reperfusion in ponies. Equine Vet J 1991;23(6):426–33.
[25] Moore RM, Bertone AL, Muir WW, et al. Histopathologic evidence of reperfusion injury in the large colon of horses after low-flow ischemia. Am J Vet Res 1994;55(10):1434–43.
[26] Mills PC, Roberts CA, Smith NC. Effects of ozone and airway inflammation on glutathione status and iron homeostasis in the lungs of horses. Am J Vet Res 1996;57(9):1359–63.
[27] Mills PC, Higgins AJ. Oxidant injury, nitric oxide and pulmonary vascular function: implications for the exercising horse. Vet J 1997;153(2):125–48.
[28] Art T, Kirschvink N, Smith N, et al. Indices of oxidative stress in blood and pulmonary epithelium lining fluid in horses suffering from recurrent airway obstruction. Equine Vet J 1999; 31(5):397–401.
[29] Kirschvink N, Art T, Smith N, et al. Effect of exercise and COPD crisis on isoprostane concentration in plasma and bronchoalveolar lavage fluid in horses. Equine Vet J Suppl 1999;30: 88–91.
[30] Kirschvink N, Smith N, Fievez L, et al. Effect of chronic airway inflammation and exercise on pulmonary and systemic antioxidant status of healthy and heaves-affected horses. Equine Vet J 2002;34(6):563–71.
[31] Kirschvink N, Art T, de Moffarts B, et al. Relationship between markers of blood oxidant status and physiologic variables in healthy and heaves-affected horses after exercise. Equine Vet J Suppl 2002;34:159–64.
[32] Kirschvink N, Bureau F, Art T, et al. Bronchoconstrictive properties of inhaled 8-epi-PGF2alpha in healthy and heaves-susceptible horses. Vet Res 2001;32(5):397–407.
[33] Art T, Kirschvink N, Smith N, et al. Cardiorespiratory measurements and indices of oxidative stress in exercising COPD horses. Equine Vet J Suppl 1999;30:83–7.
[34] Costa LR, Seahorn TL, Moore RM, et al. Plasma and bronchoalveolar fluid concentrations of nitric oxide and localization of nitric oxide synthesis in the lungs of horses with summer pasture-associated obstructive pulmonary disease. Am J Vet Res 2001;62(9):1381–6.
[35] Marlin DJ, Fenn K, Smith N, et al. Changes in circulatory antioxidant status in horses during prolonged exercise. J Nutr 2002;132(6 Suppl 2):1622S–7S.
[36] Kinnunen S, Hyyppa S, Lehmuskero A, et al. Oxygen radical absorbance capacity (ORAC) and exercise-induced oxidative stress in trotters. Eur J Appl Physiol 2005;95(5–6):550–6.
[37] Ji LL, Dillon DA, Bump KD, et al. Antioxidant enzyme response to exercise in equine erythrocytes. Equine Veterinary Science 1990;10(5):380–3.
[38] de Moffarts B, Kirschvink N, Art T, et al. Effect of oral antioxidant supplementation on blood antioxidant status in trained Thoroughbred horses. Vet J 2005;169(1):65–74.
[39] Avellini L, Chiaradia E, Gaiti A. Effect of exercise training, selenium and vitamin E on some free radical scavengers in horses (Equus caballus). Comp Biochem Physiol B Biochem Mol Biol 1999;123(2):147–54.

[40] Mills PC, Smith NC, Harris RC, et al. Effect of allopurinol on the formation of reactive oxygen species during intense exercise in the horse. Res Vet Sci 1997;62(1):11–6.
[41] Williams CA, Kronfeldt DS, Hess TM, et al. Antioxidant supplementation and subsequent oxidative stress of horses during an 80-km endurance race. J Anim Sci 2004;82(2):588–94.
[42] Hargreaves BJ, Kronfeld DS, Waldron JN, et al. Antioxidant status of horses during two 80-km endurance races. J Nutr 2002;132(6 Suppl 2):1781S–3S.
[43] Mills PC, Smith NC, Casas I, et al. Effects of exercise intensity and environmental stress on indices of oxidative stress and iron homeostasis during exercise in the horse. Eur J Appl Physiol Occup Physiol 1996;74(1–2):60–6.
[44] Chiaradia E, Avellini L, Rueca F, et al. Physical exercise, oxidative stress and muscle damage in racehorses. Comp Biochem Physiol B Biochem Mol Biol 1998;119(4):833–6.
[45] Divers TJ, Cummings JE, de Lahunta A, et al. Evaluation of the risk of motor neuron disease in horses fed a diet low in vitamin E and high in copper and iron. Am J Vet Res 2006;67(1):120–6.
[46] Divers TJ, Mohammed HO, Cummings JF, et al. Equine motor neuron disease: findings in 28 horses and proposal of a pathophysiological mechanism for the disease. Equine Vet J 1994;26(5):409–15.
[47] Polack EW, King JM, Cummings JF, et al. Concentrations of trace minerals in the spinal cord of horses with equine motor neuron disease. Am J Vet Res 2000;61(6):609–11.
[48] de la Rua-Domenech R, Wiedmann M, Mohammed HO, et al. Equine motor neuron disease is not linked to Cu/Zn superoxide dismutase mutations: sequence analysis of the equine Cu/Zn superoxide dismutase cDNA. Gene 1996;178(1–2):83–8.
[49] Kim DY, Taylor HW, Moore RM, et al. Articular chondrocyte apoptosis in equine osteoarthritis. Vet J 2003;166(1):52–7.
[50] Auer DE, Ng JC, Seawright AA. Free radical oxidation products in plasma and synovial fluid of horses with synovial inflammation. Aust Vet J 1993;70(2):49–52.
[51] Dimock AN, Siciliano PD, McIlwraith CW. Evidence supporting an increased presence of reactive oxygen species in the diseased equine joint. Equine Vet J 2000;32(5):439–43.
[52] van der Harst M, Bull S, Brama PA, et al. Nitrite and nitrotyrosine concentrations in articular cartilage, subchondral bone, and trabecular bone of normal juvenile, normal adult, and osteoarthritic adult equine metacarpophalangeal joints. J Rheumatol 2006;33(8):1662–7.
[53] McFarlane D, Dybdal N, Donaldson MT, et al. Nitration and increased alpha-synuclein expression associated with dopaminergic neurodegeneration in equine pituitary pars intermedia dysfunction. J Neuroendocrinol 2005;17(2):73–80.
[54] Keen JA, McLaren M, Chandler KJ, et al. Biochemical indices of vascular function, glucose metabolism and oxidative stress in horses with equine Cushing's disease. Equine Vet J 2004;36(3):226–9.
[55] McFarlane D, Cribb AE. Systemic and pituitary pars intermedia antioxidant capacity associated with pars intermedia oxidative stress and dysfunction in horses. Am J Vet Res 2005;66(12):2065–72.
[56] McConnico RS, Weinstock D, Poston ME, et al. Myeloperoxidase activity of the large intestine in an equine model of acute colitis. Am J Vet Res 1999;60(7):807–13.
[57] McConnico RS, Argenzio RA, Roberts MC. Prostaglandin E2 and reactive oxygen metabolite damage in the cecum in a pony model of acute colitis. Can J Vet Res 2002;66(1):50–4.
[58] Yaralioglu-Gurgoze S, Cetin H, Cen O, et al. Changes in malondialdehyde concentrations and glutathione peroxidase activity in purebred Arabian mares with endometritis. Vet J 2005;170(1):135–7.
[59] Norman TE, Chaffin MK, Johnson MC, et al. Intravascular hemolysis associated with severe cutaneous burn injuries in five horses. J Am Vet Med Assoc 2005;226(12):2039–43, 2002.
[60] McMeniman NP, Hintz HF. Effect of vitamin E status on lipid peroxidation in exercised horses. Equine Vet J 1992;24(6):482–4.

[61] Deaton CM, Marlin DJ, Smith NC, et al. Pulmonary epithelial lining fluid and plasma ascorbic acid concentrations in horses affected by recurrent airway obstruction. Am J Vet Res 2004;65(1):80–7.
[62] Deaton CM, Marlin DJ, Smith NC, et al. Pulmonary bioavailability of ascorbic acid in an ascorbate-synthesising species, the horse. Free Radic Res 2003;37(4):461–7.
[63] White A, Estrada M, Walker K, et al. Role of exercise and ascorbate on plasma antioxidant capacity in Thoroughbred race horses. Comp Biochem Physiol A Mol Integr Physiol 2001; 128(1):99–104.
[64] Deaton CM, Marlin DJ, Roberts CA, et al. Antioxidant supplementation and pulmonary function at rest and exercise. Equine Vet J Suppl 2002;34:58–65.
[65] Kirschvink N, Fievez L, Bougnet V, et al. Effect of nutritional antioxidant supplementation on systemic and pulmonary antioxidant status, airway inflammation and lung function in heaves-affected horses. Equine Vet J 2002;34(7):705–12.
[66] Deaton CM, Marlin DJ, Smith NC, et al. Antioxidant supplementation in horses affected by recurrent airway obstruction. J Nutr 2004;134(8 Suppl):2065S–7S.
[67] Rotting AK, Freeman DE, Eurell JA, et al. Effects of acetylcysteine and migration of resident eosinophils in an in vitro model of mucosal injury and restitution in equine right dorsal colon. Am J Vet Res 2003;64(10):1205–12.
[68] Lochner F, Sherban DG, Sangiah S, et al. Effects of allopurinol on endotoxin-induced increase in serum xanthine oxidase in the horse. Res Vet Sci 1990;49(1):104–9.
[69] Sullins KE, White NA, Lundin CS, et al. Prevention of ischaemia-induced small intestinal adhesions in foals. Equine Vet J 2004;36(5):370–5.
[70] Vatistas NJ, Snyder JR, Hildebrand SV, et al. Effects of the 21-aminosteroid U-74389G on ischemia and reperfusion injury of the ascending colon in horses. Am J Vet Res 1993;54(12):2155–60.
[71] Vatistas NJ, Snyder JR, Hildebrand SV, et al. Effects of U-74389G, a novel 21-aminosteroid, on small intestinal ischemia and reperfusion injury in horses. Am J Vet Res 1996;57(5):762–70.
[72] Dabareiner RM, White NA III, Donaldson L. Evaluation of Carolina rinse solution as a treatment for ischaemia reperfusion of the equine jejunum. Equine Vet J 2003;35(7):642–6.
[73] Young BL, White NA, Donaldson LL, et al. Treatment of ischaemic jejunum with topical and intraluminal Carolina rinse. Equine Vet J 2002;34(5):469–74.
[74] Van Hoogmoed LM, Snyder JR, Nieto J, et al. In vitro evaluation of a customized solution for use in attenuating effects of ischemia and reperfusion in the equine small intestine. Am J Vet Res 2001;62(11):1679–86.
[75] Van Hoogmoed LM, Nieto JE, Snyder JR, et al. In vitro evaluation of an intraluminal solution to attenuate effects of ischemia and reperfusion in the small intestine of horses. Am J Vet Res 2002;63(10):1389–94.
[76] Singh RK, Kooreman KM, Babbs CF, et al. Potential use of simple manganese salts as antioxidant drugs in horses. Am J Vet Res 1992;53(10):1822–9.

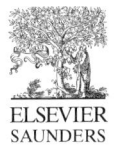

Neonatal Foal Resuscitation
Jonathan E. Palmer, VMD[a,b,c],*

[a]Section of Large Animal Medicine, School of Veterinary Medicine, University of Pennsylvania, 382 West Street Road, Kennett Square, PA 19348, USA
[b]Section of Anesthesia, Emergency and Critical Care Medicine, School of Veterinary Medicine, New Bolton Center, University of Pennsylvania, 382 West Street Road, Kennett Square, PA 19348, USA
[c]Graham French Neonatal Section, Connelly Intensive Care Unit, New Bolton Center, University of Pennsylvania, 382 West Street Road, Kennett Square, PA 19348, USA

There are many reasons for cardiopulmonary arrest in foals. Usually, it is secondary to other systemic conditions, such as septic shock or respiratory failure, and not attributable to primary cardiac failure. Often, the inciting condition is progressive and is treatable in the early stages; however, if left to its natural course, it eventually leads to respiratory arrest and then bradycardia, which deteriorates to asystole. Unlike human adults, in whom the principal cause of cardiopulmonary failure is coronary artery disease, ventricular fibrillation (VF) is not a common presenting arrhythmia. Early recognition and treatment of the predisposing condition can often prevent the arrest. Birth is a high-risk period, because neonates may fail the transition from fetal to neonatal physiology. Prompt intervention is vital in these cases.

The most important step in resuscitation is thorough preparation. At the moment of crisis, there is no time to formulate a plan. Well-conceived algorithms must be initiated once the nature of the crisis is recognized (Fig. 1). Airway equipment and emergency drugs must be organized in a manner that allows them to be easily transported stall side. In the hospital setting, this can be accomplished by organizing a "crash cart." In ambulatory practice, organizing the equipment in grips can be helpful. Printed algorithms with drug doses in terms of amounts in milliliters needed for the typical foal should also be readily available (Table 1). In the discussion elsewhere in this article, techniques ranging from basic to advanced life support are outlined in an effort to prepare the practitioner to meet the challenge of the moment of crisis with tools that result in a successful outcome.

* University of Pennsylvania, New Bolton Center, 382 West Street Road, Kennett Square, PA 19348.
 E-mail address: jepalmer@vet.upenn.edu

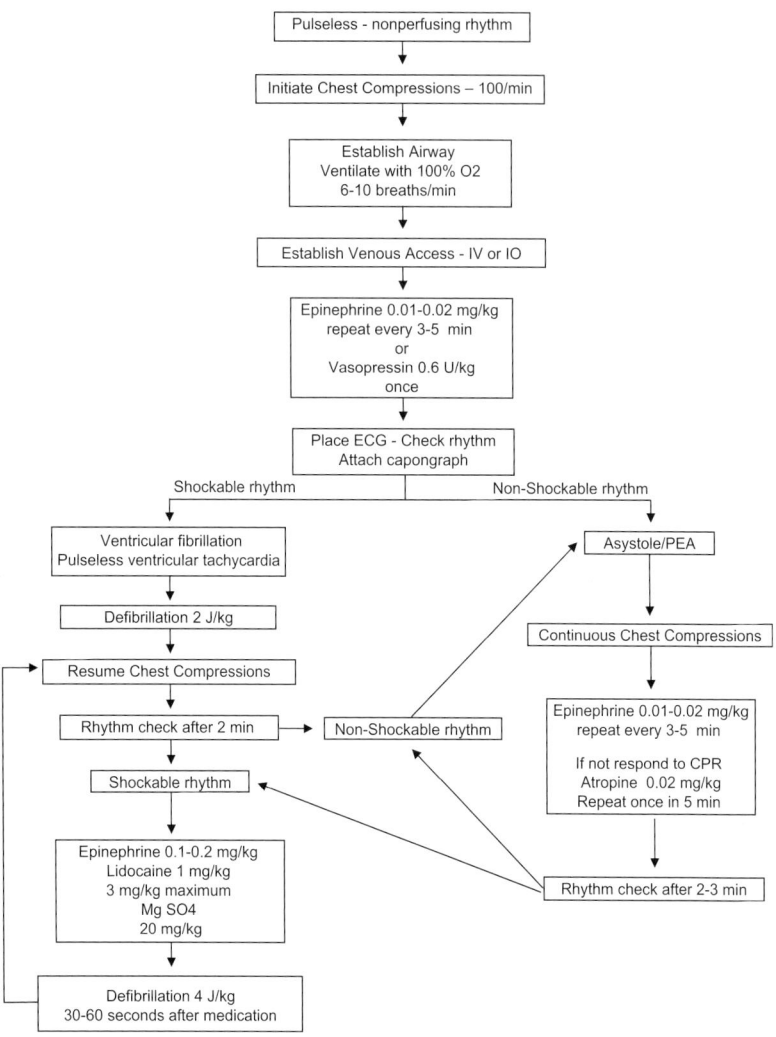

Fig. 1. Management of cardiac arrest.

Reasons for cardiopulmonary failure

Pulseless cardiac arrest may be produced by any one of four rhythms: VF, pulseless ventricular tachycardia (VT), pulseless electrical activity (PEA), or asystole [1]. VF or VT is a rare presenting arrhythmia in cardiac failure in foals, because primary cardiac failure is an unusual reason for cardiac arrest. When primary cardiac failure occurs, it is usually secondary to hypoxic-ischemic or cytokine-mediated myocardial damage, congenital cardiac defects, myocarditis, or endocarditis with coronary artery embolism.

Table 1
Dosage (mL/kg) of drugs commonly used in cardiopulmonary resuscitation

Drug	Dose (per kg)	Supplied	mL/kg	mL/20 kg	mL/30 kg	mL/40 kg	mL/50 kg	mL/60 kg	mL/70 kg
Epinephrine, low dose	0.01–0.02 mg	1 mg/mL	0.01–0.02	0.2–0.4, 3–5 min	0.3–0.6, 3–5 min	0.4–0.8, 3–5 min	0.5–1, 3–5 min	0.6–1.2, 3–5 min	0.7–1.4, 3–5 min
Epinephrine, high dose	0.1 mg	1 mg/mL	0.1	2, 3–5 min	3, 3–5 min	4, 3–5 min	5, 3–5 min	6, 3–5 min	7, 3–5 min
Vasopressin	0.6 U	20 U/mL	0.03	0.6	0.9	1.2	1.5	1.8	2
Lidocaine	1.5 mg	2%	0.075	1.6	2.25	3	3.75	4.5	5.25
				Every 5 minutes to maximum dose of 3 mg/kg			Every 5 minutes to maximum dose of 3 mg/kg		
Atropine	0.02 mg	20 mg/mL	0.001	0.8, maximum of 2 times	1.1, maximum of 2 times	1.5, maximum of 2 times	1.8, maximum of 2 times	2.2, maximum of 2 times	2.6, maximum of 2 times
CaCl	20 mg (CaCl)	10% CaCl	0.2	4	6	8	10	12	14
Mg SO$_4$	25–50 mg/kg	50%, 500 mg/mL	0.05–0.1	1–2	1.5–3	2–4	2.5–5	3–6	3.5–7

Abbreviations: CaCl, calcium chloride; Mg SO$_4$, magnesium sulfate.

Cardiopulmonary failure in foals usually occurs secondary to systemic disease. Systemic disease may cause secondary respiratory or cardiac failure leading to hypoxic acidosis. The hypoxic acidosis, in turn, causes respiratory arrest, followed by development of a nonperfusing bradycardia, PEA, and, finally, asystole. If resuscitation is begun before a nonperfusing cardiac rhythm develops, the likelihood of revival is good (survival rate as high as 50%). If resuscitation efforts are delayed until after development of asystole, however, a less than 10% survival rate is to be expected. Because the cause of arrest in most cases is systemic disease and the onset of arrest follows progressive respiratory and circulatory failure, with careful attention to development of signs, resuscitation can be begun before complete failure occurs.

Common causes of secondary cardiopulmonary arrest include perinatal hypoxia leading to central respiratory center damage, resulting in hypoventilation; primary lung disease leading to hypoventilation and hypoxia; septic shock; hypovolemia; metabolic acidosis; hyperkalemia (eg, ruptured bladder); vasovagal reflex; hypoglycemia; and hypothermia. Less common causes include cardiac tamponade, tension pneumothorax, and trauma. To save the patient, the underlying cause of the arrest must be recognized and treated. Cardiopulmonary resuscitation (CPR) may revive the patient; however, without addressing the underlying cause, repeated cardiopulmonary arrest is likely. Also, if the underlying cause cannot be cured, it is inhumane to perform CPR because it may prolong suffering needlessly.

Recognition of impending failure may be straightforward; however, at times, it can be difficult when only relying on physical findings. Respiratory failure is marked by hypercapnia and hypoxia caused by inadequate ventilation. Foals with failure attributable to respiratory center damage secondary to peripartum asphyxia, fetal inflammatory response syndrome (FIRS), or neonatal systemic inflammatory response syndrome (SIRS) do not sense the hypoxia or hypercapnia, and thus have an inadequate respiratory effort. Although some may have abnormal respiratory patterns secondary to central disease, such as periodic apnea, most have an apparently normal respiratory rate and minimal effort, making their respiratory failure difficult to recognize.

Failure secondary to intrinsic lung disease, airway obstruction, or fatigue results in progressive respiratory failure that is easily recognized. In these cases, signs of respiratory compensation precede failure. Signs include increased respiratory rate (tachypnea), increased respiratory depth (hyperpnea), increased work of breathing, nostril flare, use of accessory respiratory muscles, and sinus tachycardia. When a foal with these signs has what seems to be rapid improvement, it may, in fact, be fatigue or toxic effects of extreme hypercapnia and prolonged hypoxia preceding respiratory arrest.

Septic shock can lead to cardiopulmonary arrest. Respiratory failure and shock may begin as distinct problems but progress in concert to cardiopulmonary failure. There is a dynamic balance between the oxygen content of blood and cardiac output. If either falls, the other must increase to ensure adequate oxygen delivery to the tissues. Oxygen content can only increase marginally when breathing room air. Any significant decrease in cardiac output results in decreased oxygen delivery unless oxygen content is increased by increasing the concentration of inspired oxygen with intranasal oxygen.

Cardiopulmonary failure leads inevitably to cardiopulmonary arrest. Signs of cardiopulmonary failure include tachycardia, depression (nonresponsiveness), oliguria, hypotonia, a weak proximal pulse with a weak or absent peripheral pulse, and prolonged capillary refill time (CRT). Late ominous signs include bradycardia, hypotension, an irregular respiratory pattern, and paradoxical respiration (wave-chest respiratory pattern).

Clinical approach to cardiopulmonary resuscitation

When cardiopulmonary arrest is caused by primary cardiac failure, the priority is initiation of cardiac compressions. Ventilation is much less important and should not be pursued if it means delaying or interrupting cardiac compressions. Conversely, when cardiopulmonary arrest is caused by systemic disease initiating pulmonary failure and leading to cardiac failure, ventilation is more important. In such cases, if there is at least a minimally perfusing bradycardia when the crisis is recognized, ventilation should be established before any other action is taken. Delaying cardiac contractions in the first case or delaying ventilation in the second case significantly decreases the chances of successful resuscitation [2]. Although the priority, and thus order of initiation, may differ depending on the circumstances, the steps necessary for successful CPR include establishing an airway, ventilation, chest compressions, administering drugs, determining the cardiac arrhythmia, and treating accordingly.

Establishing an airway

When an endotracheal tube is not immediately available, mouth-to-nose ventilation can be effective, facilitated by the fact that foals are obligate nasal breathers. This can be achieved by placing the fingers of one hand just behind the foal's chin with the palm and thumb occluding the down nostril and placing the other hand on the foal's poll so that the head can be maximally dorsiflexed, straightening the airway, and thus decreasing the possibility of aerophagia. Alternately, the foal's head can be turned so that the poll is on the ground, resulting in maximal dorsiflexion, allowing the free hand to place pressure on the cricoid to ensure occlusion of the esophagus. The foal's head should not be elevated because this may further compromise cerebral circulation. While breathing into the up nostril, the chest can be observed to rise, ensuring the proper tidal volume. The fractional inspired oxygen content of exhaled air is approximately 16% to 18%, but this is adequate when perfusion is failing.

As soon as an endotracheal tube is available, it should be placed. A cuffed endotracheal tube 55 cm in length works well for nasotracheal intubation in the foal. The largest endotracheal tube that fits should be used to minimize its resistance. In the average Thoroughbred or Standardbred foal, a 9-mm internal diameter works well. Small-breed foals (eg, Arabians) may require a 7- to 8-mm tube, whereas large foals may require a 10- to 12-mm tube. Whenever possible, sterile technique should be used to avoid introduction of nosocomial pathogens; however, because time is of the essence, the first priority is rapid intubation and initiation of resuscitation. Nasotracheal intubation can be performed without assistance in cardiopulmonary failure, allowing others present to begin cardiac compressions, establish intravenous access, prepare appropriate drug dosages, or attach monitoring equipment. It should be performed with the foal in lateral recumbency so that cardiac compressions can be begun without delay. Do not elevate the foal's head because this further compromises cerebral blood flow. Dorsiflex the foal's head to straighten the airway. Pass the endotracheal tube through the nasal passage. Once the tube reaches the level of the arytenoids, a twisting motion facilitates passage by allowing the beveled end to spread the arytenoids. If it is in the trachea, the tube should advance with little or no resistance. Palpate the esophagus to ensure proper placement. Inadvertent inflation of the stomach is clearly detrimental. Advance the endotracheal tube until only the adapter is visible at the nostril to minimize dead space. Secure with ties to a halter or around the poll. Inflate the cuff to ensure a seal (fill the cuff until no air leak is heard during positive-pressure ventilation).

Ventilation

A self-inflating bag-valve device designed for human adult resuscitation (1600 mL with a 2600-mL oxygen reservoir bag) is easy to use, versatile, and safe. The bag draws room air if no other gas source is available; however, when it is attached to an oxygen source, high concentrations of oxygen can be delivered. The reservoir should be kept full to maintain high concentrations. The flow needed to maintain the reservoir depends on the minute volume being delivered. If the self-inflating bag has a pop-off valve (usually set to 35–45 cm of water to avoid barotrauma during normal ventilation), it needs to be easily occluded when low lung compliance, high airway resistance, an endotracheal tube obstructed by secretions or kinks, or the presence of pneumothorax makes high airway pressures necessary.

It has recently been realized that ventilation can negatively affect the outcome in CPR [3]. Increased thoracic pressure induced by positive-pressure ventilation interferes significantly with cardiac return and decreases coronary and cerebral perfusion [4]. Recognition of this cardiocerebral-pulmonary interaction during CPR has resulted in a reassessment of previous recommendations for ventilation during CPR. When primary cardiac arrest is the reason for CPR and respiratory function was normal until the arrest, the negative aspects of ventilation outweigh the positive affects and ventilation should be pursued secondarily and minimally at first. When, as in most neonates, there is asphyxial arrest (respiratory failure precedes cardiac arrest), the positive aspects of ventilation become more important to survival. During CPR, cardiac output is no better than 25% to 30% of normal [2]. Intrapulmonary shunting, which occurs during CPR, further decreases effective alveolar perfusion. This means that the amount of ventilation needed for ideal matching with the perfusion is much less than the normal minute volume [3]. Trying to maintain the normal minute volume using a normal respiratory rate and tidal volumes does not help to increase gas exchange in light of the limited perfusion, and the resultant negative effect of increased time of positive thoracic pressure, in fact, decreases the cardiac output further. Thus, although prearrest and postarrest normal tidal volume and respiratory rate with oxygen-enriched gas are important, during CPR, tidal volume and rate should be limited. The inhaled gas should be 100% oxygen to maximize loading of all matched perfusion [2]. Inspiration should be limited to no more than 1 second, and the respiratory rate should be limited to no more than 8 to 10 breaths per minute [2]. If an endotracheal tube has been placed, ventilation does not need to be coordinated with chest compressions. The goal should be rapid infrequent breaths. It is helpful to place a watch with a second hand in view of whoever is ventilating the foal, with instructions to give no more than 1 rapid breath every 10 seconds (although if this were strictly done, the rate would be 6 breaths per minute; inevitably, during the stress of CPR, the rate is likely to be more rapid, but this technique should help to limit the rate). Careful observation of chest excursion is the best way to gauge tidal volume, with the knowledge that the goal is not a deep breath. Auscultation of the lung fields after endotracheal placement and initiation of ventilation to ensure even air flow can be helpful but should not be done at the expense of other vital CPR procedures.

Cardiac compressions

Chest compressions should be initiated immediately, if a nonperfusing cardiac rhythm is present. Do not delay until cardiac contractions stop. The mechanism of blood flow during chest compression is not clear [5]. The cardiac pump theory suggests that chest pressure causes cardiac compression, propelling blood with cardiac valves directing the blood flow forward. The thoracic pump theory suggests that the increased thoracic pressure caused by the compression propels the blood and that the venous valves direct it forward, whereas noncompliant cardiac valves (as a result of myocardial rigor) make the cardiac contribution to blood flow minimal. No matter how compression propels blood, it has become clear that during the recoil of the chest wall between compressions, the resulting negative intrathoracic pressure is important in producing venous return. The goal should be a rate of 100 compressions, with complete chest recoil between compressions. The mantra has become "push hard, push fast" [6]. It is equally important to minimize interruptions in compression, with a maximum interruption of 10 seconds. Longer interruptions with the accompanying failure of coronary perfusion are an important cause of failure to return to spontaneous circulation. All interruptions, such as those that might occur during efforts to intubate, rhythm checks, or defibrillation, should be well planned, coordinated whenever possible, and minimized to less than 10 seconds, with at least 2 minutes of chest compressions between interruptions [2,5].

Cardiac compression can be done by placing the foal on a firm surface (remove any bedding under foal) and positioning the foal with its withers against a wall so that it does not move during forceful compressions. Time is of the essence, and it should not be wasted by unnecessarily repositioning the foal. While kneeling between the foal's front and hind legs, place the palm of the hand with the fist closed over the foal's heart. Place the other hand on top of the first to reinforce the compressing hand. The elbows should remain straight, and the motion for compression should originate from the waist (with the upper body weight powering the compression, resulting in increased endurance). Chest compression results in no more than 25% to 30% of normal cardiac output. To maximize cardiac output, at least half of the duty cycle should be relaxation. This is easiest to achieve with a rapid compression rate of approximately 100 per minute. The resuscitator should not be overly ambitious in setting a rate. Too rapid a rate results in early operator fatigue. If an airway is secured, coordination between ventilation and chest compression is not needed.

Methods for measuring effectiveness of cardiac output

Central arterial pulse (femoral or carotid artery) has been used traditionally as an assessment of effectiveness of the chest compressions. Myocardial blood flow does not depend on the palpated arterial systolic pressure, however, and retrograde blood flow into the venous system may produce femoral vein pulsations. Palpation of a pulse in the femoral triangle may indicate venous rather than arterial blood flow. Carotid pulsations during CPR do not indicate the efficacy of coronary blood flow or myocardial or cerebral perfusion during CPR. Although the lack of a palpable pulse during CPR may indicate inadequate forward flow, the degree of forward flow cannot be estimated accurately in the presence of a palpable pulse, because pressures generated may be transmitted equally to the venous and arterial vasculatures [7-9]. Attempting to palpate pulses during CPR is a waste of effort.

Monitoring pupil size is an indirect indication of adequate cerebral perfusion. When perfusion of the head becomes inadequate, the pupils dilate widely. When chest compression results in adequate perfusion to the head, the pupils assume a more neutral size. Pupil size can be monitored by the same person who is performing the chest compressions. The chest compression technique should be adjusted as indicated by pupil size.

The most effective measurement of cardiac output during CPR is end-tidal carbon dioxide (P_{ETCO_2}). When there is no cardiac output to the lungs, the P_{ETCO_2} is 0 (alveoli are ventilated but not perfused). When chest compression results in effective cardiac output and lung perfusion occurs, the P_{ETCO_2} increases. As cardiac output increases with effective the chest compressions, the P_{ETCO_2} increases to a level of 12 to 18 mm Hg. Although the P_{ETCO_2} level correlates well with cardiac output, there are some manipulations during CPR that can cause a change in the P_{ETCO_2} independent of cardiac output. High-dose epinephrine therapy can cause a transient decrease in the P_{ETCO_2}, and treatment with bicarbonate can increase the P_{ETCO_2} (buffering of acid in the central venous system results in a higher concentration of carbon dioxide in the blood delivered to the lungs). Capnography results in immediate feedback to the resuscitator, allowing for beat-to-beat modification of technique, ensuring that the most effective cardiac output is achieved. Arterial blood gas (ABG) and pulse oximetry are not useful monitors of the effectiveness of CPR [9].

Vascular access

Establishing vascular access is essential if the neonate does not respond immediately to chest compressions and ventilation. Many patients already have an intravenous catheter in place, because cardiopulmonary failure in neonates is usually secondary to other serious systemic diseases. For those that do not, the jugular vein should be catheterized using whatever available materials the resuscitator believes are likely to result in the most rapid vascular access.

Drugs can be given by the intratracheal route, but absorption is poor; thus, this route should only be used if there are no other possibilities. Low-volume lipid-soluble drugs, such as epinephrine, atropine, lidocaine, and naloxone, have been shown to be absorbed. The drug must be delivered beyond the endotracheal tube into the bronchial tree. This can be accomplished by passing infusion tubing down the endotracheal tube and chasing the drug with fluids. An equally effective and more expedient method involves transtracheal injection of the drugs. This can be achieved by first identifying the level of the inflated cuff on the endotracheal tube by palpation, placing a needle below the level of the tube (usually close to the thoracic inlet) perpendicular to the skin between tracheal rings into the tracheal lumen, injecting the drug, chasing the drug with air in the syringe, and following the injection with a breath. Drugs given by this route are not reliably absorbed. If epinephrine is given by this route, the dose should be 0.1 mg/kg or more (larger than the intravenous dose). Pulmonary tissue may act as a reservoir for the drug, leading to prolonged absorption during the postarrest resuscitation period, possibly causing significant problems [9].

A more useful circulatory access route when vascular access is not immediately available is the intraosseous route [10–13]. Drugs injected into the bone marrow are absorbed almost immediately into the systemic circulation. The marrow cavity does not collapse in the presence of hypovolemia or profound peripheral circulatory shock; thus, venous return is more likely to be maintained. The pharmacodynamics of intraosseous infused drugs are almost the same as those for intravenous infusion [14]. Drugs that can be administered by the intraosseous route include fluids, glucose, sodium bicarbonate, calcium chloride (CaCl), blood, plasma, epinephrine, lidocaine, atropine, dopamine, dobutamine, vasopressin, antimicrobials, phenobarbital, diazepam, butorphanol, insulin, mannitol, and virtually any drug that can be administered intravenously [15–18].

The technique that this author uses for intraosseous needle placement is as follows. The entry point is the proximal tibia on the midline of the anterior medial flat surface 2 to 4 cm below the proximal tibial physis. Care must be taken to be well below the physis to ensure entering the marrow. This site is preferred because of the lack of soft tissue structures over the bone, rapid identification of the landmarks, flat entry surface, and ease of penetrating the marrow. It is well away from areas occupied by other resuscitators. Stabilization after entry may be difficult at this site because of the medial location. If the patient is unconscious, it is not necessary to use local anesthetics, thus speeding vascular access. Aseptically prepare the site if time allows. A stab incision is usually necessary to prevent interference caused by the skin wrapping around the needle as it is turned.

In mature newborn foals, standard intraosseous needles designed for human adults can be used (12-gauge 2.3-cm intraosseous infusion needle; Sur-Fast Intraosseous Infusion Needle, Cook Critical Care, Bloomington, Indiana). In premature foals, twins, and foals with intrauterine growth restriction that have incomplete ossification, a 16- to 18-gauge spinal needle can be used but does pose a danger of bending or breaking because of its length and narrow gauge. The needle should be placed with a screwing action directed distally at a slight angle ($10°–15°$ from vertical) while applying firm downward pressure until a release is felt as the needle enters the marrow. The needle should stand without support. Fluid should easily flow through the needle without resistance when flushed. The ability to infuse fluids easily through conventional infusion tubing with no extravasation confirms correct placement. The needle and infusion line should be secured in such a way that the site can be observed for extravasation of fluids indicating improper placement. Avoid placing the needle where the cortex has already been perforated (unsuccessful placement attempt or fracture). Failed attempts with cortical perforation require moving to a new site. Complications include extravasation into subcutaneous tissues, incomplete insertion of needle, and overpenetration through the opposite cortex. Cellulitis associated with extravasation is uncommon, as is osteomyelitis. Growth plate injury does not seem to be a problem [10].

Drug therapy

In general drugs used during CPR are unsupported or poorly supported by strong evidence [1]. Some are used by long tradition and experience, and others are used because of physiologic rationale or inference from their action in similar pathophysiologic settings. Most randomized controlled clinical trials have failed to show clear survival benefits, in part, because of the poor outcome in all cases of cardiac arrest. There have been no studies of CPR in foals, and all information about drugs and doses as well as all other aspects of CPR is based on experience and extrapolation from other species.

Epinephrine

Epinephrine is an endogenous catecholamine with α- and β-adrenergic effects, but it is the α-adrenergic effects that are most helpful in cardiac resuscitation. Epinephrine can improve coronary perfusion pressure during cardiac arrest. During chest compressions, coronary blood flow is restricted to the diastolic period. Diastolic aortic pressure determines coronary perfusion, because during cardiac arrest, there is no coronary capillary resistance and central venous pressure is low because of minimal venous return. Epinephrine's α-adrenergic effects increase diastolic aortic pressure by simultaneously preventing runoff into peripheral tissues (by peripheral arterial constriction) and increasing aortic tone. The combination of effective chest compressions and the action of epinephrine results in a return of coronary perfusion, which is the most important step in resolving cardiac arrest no matter what the cause. Without coronary perfusion, there is no hope of return to a normal cardiac rhythm. The value and safety of the β-adrenergic effects of epinephrine are controversial because they may increase myocardial work and reduce myocardial perfusion [15,16].

Beneficial and toxic physiologic effects of epinephrine administration during CPR have been shown. Low-dose (0.01–0.02 mg/kg) and high-dose (0.1 mg/kg) regimens have been proposed. Although a return to spontaneous circulation may occur more commonly with the high-dose regimen, the secondary toxic effects seem to make survival less likely [1,17–19]. Anecdotal experience in foals suggests that myocardial necrosis is more extensive with high-dose therapy. Although there may be some cases that could benefit from the high-dose regimen, it should not be used routinely.

Epinephrine therapy is indicated for cardiac arrest regardless of the underlying cause or rhythm. It is appropriate to administer a 0.01- to 0.02-mg/kg dose of epinephrine intravenously or intraosseously every 3 minutes. Higher doses may be indicated to treat specific cases. If intravenous or intraosseous access is delayed or cannot be established, epinephrine may be given by the endotracheal route at a dose of 0.05 to 0.1 mg/kg. Complications include increased cardiac oxygen demand with myocardial necrosis and post-resuscitation hypertension with tachyarrhythmias. Epinephrine, as with all adrenergic drugs, is inactivated when mixed with bicarbonate.

Vasopressin

Vasopressin is a nonadrenergic endogenous stress hormone that is a potent peripheral vasoconstrictor. Its vasoconstrictor action is more potent than that of angiotensin II or norepinephrine, but its pressor action is minimal in normal individuals because of baroreceptor-mediated bradycardia, which prevents pressure increase. The pressor activity of vasopressin is marked in cardiac arrest [9].

Vasopressin has been found to be as effective as epinephrine, no matter what the presenting nonperfusing cardiac rhythm, in aiding return to spontaneous circulation. There is some evidence that when the nonperfusing rhythm is asystole, the use of vasopressin or vasopressin in combination with epinephrine may be more effective than epinephrine alone in returning spontaneous circulation [20,21].

Vasopressin can be used in all causes of cardiac arrest. The dose of vasopressin for pulseless cardiac arrest is a total of 0.6 U/kg given as a single dose or divided. Because the effect lasts 10 to 20 minutes, repeat doses are unnecessary. Postresuscitation hypertension or arrhythmias are not likely.

Atropine

Atropine sulfate can reverse cholinergic-mediated decreases in heart rate, systemic vascular resistance, and blood pressure. PEA, which encompasses a heterogeneous group of pulseless rhythms that includes pseudo–electromechanical dissociation (pseudo-EMD), idioventricular rhythms, ventricular escape rhythms, postdefibrillation idioventricular rhythms, and bradyasystolic rhythms, may respond to atropine. Asystole can be precipitated or exacerbated by excessive vagal tone; thus, administration of atropine is consistent with a physiologic approach [1].

High vagal tone (except secondary to hypoxia) is an uncommon cause of the initial bradycardia that becomes PEA in neonatal foals. Neonatal bradycardia is generally caused by hypoxia and should be treated initially by hyperventilation with 100% oxygen and epinephrine if it becomes pulseless. Early treatment with atropine may exacerbate the hypoxic insult by increasing the heart rate, resulting in a higher oxygen demand of cardiac muscle in the face of inadequate oxygen delivery. Hypoxemia and hypercapnia result in stimulation of the carotid body, increasing vagal tone with secondary bradycardia. Ventilation can correct this form of vagal-mediated bradycardia, because lung inflation stimulates the pulmonary receptors that can override the carotid body stimulus. If ventilation does not result in resolution of the bradycardia and the rhythm becomes pulseless, atropine therapy is indicated. Excessive vagal tone leading to bradyarrhythmia can be associated with gastrointestinal disease, especially when extreme intestinal distention is present. In all cases of bradycardia, atropine should not be given before chest compressions and ventilation are initiated.

In pulseless cardiac arrest associated with PEA or asystole that does not respond to ventilation, cardiac compressions, and epinephrine or vasopressin, treatment with atropine is appropriate. The atropine dose should be 0.02 mg/kg repeated once in 5 minutes if necessary. Potential complications include tachycardia leading to exacerbation of hypoxic insult by increasing the oxygen demand of cardiac muscle. Paradoxically, atropine at low doses can exacerbate bradycardia [22,23].

Lidocaine

Lidocaine is a traditional antiarrhythmic drug of long-standing and widespread familiarity, with fewer immediate side effects than may be encountered with other antiarrhythmic drugs. Its use for ventricular arrhythmias is supported by experimental studies and its use in suppressing premature ventricular contractions and preventing VF after acute myocardial infarction [24–26]. Lidocaine is thought to suppress ventricular arrhythmias by decreasing automaticity. Its local anesthetic properties may suppress ventricular ectopy. It decreases conduction of re-entrant pathways. It may reduce the disparity in action potential duration between ischemic and normal tissue. It prolongs conduction and refractoriness in ischemic tissue. It has been largely replaced in human medicine by amiodarone. As with most other resuscitation drugs, it has no proven short-term or long-term efficacy in cardiac arrest but still should be an appropriate treatment for VF or pulseless VT [1].

The initial dose is 1 mg/kg administered intravenously. If VF or pulseless VT persists, additional doses of 0.5 to 0.75 mg/kg administered by intravenous push may be administered at 5- to 10-minute intervals, to a maximum dose of 3 mg/kg. After a 1-mg/kg loading dose, a constant rate infusion (CRI) of 20 to 50 µg/kg/min may be useful in neonates. Toxic effects generally consist of neurologic signs, such as depression, paresthesia, muscle twitching, seizures, myocardial depression, and circulatory depression. Other than seizure-like activity, these signs are not evident while treating cardiac arrest. Great care needs to be taken in avoiding toxicity, because neonatal foals seem to be extremely susceptible.

Magnesium

Magnesium can be effective in terminating a torsades de pointes pattern of VF. Magnesium is unlikely to be effective in terminating irregular or polymorphic VT. The dose for torsades de pointes is 25 to 50 mg/kg diluted to 10 mL in 5% dextrose in water administered as an intravenous or intraosseous push over 5 to 20 minutes. When torsades de pointes is present in a patient with pulses, the dose may be given more slowly (over 60 minutes intravenously or intraosseously). The major side effect is hypotension when the dose is given too rapidly [1,27,28].

Fluids

Large volumes of fluids are important in treating hypovolemic or septic shock, which frequently leads to cardiac arrest. After cardiac arrest, fluid administration is contraindicated. A nonperfusing rhythm produces a situation resembling congestive heart failure, with ineffective cardiac output. With effective chest compressions, the cardiac output is only 25% to 30% of normal. If fluids are given rapidly, the venous pressure rises, impeding coronary perfusion and return of a normal cardiac rhythm, despite effective chest compressions and doses of epinephrine. If volume replacement is indicated because of severe dehydration, bolus administration is preferred rather than a continuous high flow rate. A low fluid rate should be used until spontaneous cardiac rhythm returns.

Once a perfusing rhythm returns, increased fluid rates may be needed to help maintain cardiac output. Severe hypoglycemia can lead to cardiac arrest; however, glucose-containing fluids should be avoided during resuscitation unless a patient-side glucose determination indicates severe hypoglycemia. Hyperglycemia and hyperosmolality, secondary to rapid glucose infusion, during resuscitation are associated with a poor neurologic outcome [10,25–31].

Sodium bicarbonate

The use of sodium bicarbonate during cardiac arrest remains controversial. There are few data to support its use and many contraindications. There is no evidence that bicarbonate improves the likelihood of resolution of fibrillation or survival rates. Many adverse effects have been attributed to bicarbonate therapy during cardiac arrest. Bicarbonate compromises cerebral perfusion pressure by reducing systemic vascular resistance. It can create extracellular alkalosis that shifts the oxyhemoglobin saturation curve and inhibits oxygen release. It can produce hypernatremia that results in hyperosmolality and, in human neonates, cerebral hemorrhages. It results in production of excess carbon dioxide, which diffuses into myocardial and cerebral cells, producing intracellular acidosis. It can exacerbate central venous acidosis and inactivate simultaneously administered adrenergic drugs, negating their effect [32,33].

Indications for bicarbonate administration include hyperkalemia (secondary to a ruptured bladder), preexisting metabolic acidosis leading to arrest, or phenobarbital overdose. More controversial indications include prolonged nonresponsive cardiac arrest and after return of spontaneous circulation. Hypoxic lactic acidosis is a clear contraindication.

When bicarbonate is used for special indications, an initial dose of 1 mEq/kg is recommended. Whenever possible, bicarbonate therapy should be guided by blood gas analysis or laboratory measurement.

Calcium

Calcium ions play a critical role in myocardial contractile performance; at one time, calcium was used during CPR. Retrospective and prospective studies have shown no benefit from calcium administration, however. In addition, the high serum calcium levels induced by calcium treatment may speed cell death. Calcium should not be used routinely to support circulation in the setting of cardiac arrest. When hyperkalemia, hypermagnesemia, or ionized hypocalcemia has led to cardiac arrest, however, its use is indicated [34–38].

When indicated, 10% CaCl at a dose of 20 mg/kg (0.2 mL/kg) or 23% Ca gluconate (2.14% elemental Ca) at a dose of 20 mg/kg (0.9 mL/kg) should be used. CaCl may increase bioavailability and is preferred [39]. Calcium solutions should be infused slowly.

Electrical defibrillation

Defibrillators are manual or automated, with monophasic or biphasic waveforms. Monophasic waveform defibrillators are older models that deliver current of one polarity. All currently sold defibrillators produce a biphasic waveform. There is no evidence that one waveform is more likely to result in the return of spontaneous circulation or survival, but biphasic shocks allow less energy, and thus may be safer. There is no evidence about what energy first shock is most effective or what pattern of energy levels per shock (fixed or escalating energy) is best. Automated external defibrillators (AEDs) are sophisticated and reliable computerized devices with voice prompts and the ability to evaluate the rhythm, recommend defibrillation, and automatically set all parameters. Newer models even record the frequency and depth of chest compressions and prompt for improved chest compression technique [40–43].

Defibrillation is the definitive treatment for VF and pulseless VT. Defibrillation should not be used to treat asystole or bradyarrhythmias. Ventilation with 100% oxygen and chest compressions should be continued until the moment of defibrillation. Cardiac compressions should be resumed as soon after the shock as possible to minimize the period without compressions. A rhythm check should not be done right away. Defibrillation results in depolarization of a critical mass of myocardial cells to allow spontaneous organized myocardial depolarization. Defibrillation requires electrical current to pass through the heart. The amount of current delivered to the heart depends on the energy delivered from the paddles and the transthoracic resistance [28,40].

There are numerous determinants of current flow through the heart. The largest paddles or self-adhering electrodes that fit on the chest wall leave at least 3 cm between the paddles. A paddle should be placed on each side of the chest after shaving the area. The electrode–chest wall interface can be gel pads, electrode cream, paste, or self-adhesive monitoring-defibrillation pads. Do not use saline, alcohol, ultrasound gel, or bare paddles [28].

When defibrillating, the initial charge should be 2 J/kg delivered as soon after diagnosing a shockable rhythm as possible. Subsequent defibrillations should be 4 J/kg delivered 30 to 60 seconds after treatment with epinephrine or lidocaine. There should be at least 2 minutes of chest compressions between each shock. Delivering more than one shock in a row is less likely to help and is outweighed by the harm done by the prolonged period without cardiac compressions that repeat shocks would necessitate [28,41,44].

Defibrillation is potentially dangerous to the operator and other personnel. No one should attempt defibrillation until he or she is trained in the technique and on the defibrillator being used. Improper placement of the paddles or a poor paddle-chest interface can cause serious burns. Use of alcohol before defibrillation is a fire hazard.

Management of cardiac arrest

When a pulseless cardiac rhythm is identified in a foal, the first priority should be to begin cardiac compressions. That should be followed by establishing an airway and beginning ventilation. Next, vascular access should be established. Drug therapy with epinephrine or vasopressin should follow. Monitoring equipment (eg, electrocardiography [ECG], capnography) should then be attached. The cardiac rhythm should be established as shockable (VF or pulseless VT) or nonshockable (PEA or asystole). At this point, the scheme should branch with a defibrillation, epinephrine, or lidocaine path or a continued CPR, epinephrine, or possible atropine path. The cardiac rhythm should be periodically monitored, because the scheme followed may change from one branch to the other at any time (see Fig. 1).

Postresuscitation support

The postresuscitation period is critical. Continued evaluation of cardiopulmonary function is vital, even if the foal is easily resuscitated and its condition initially seems stable. Foals often experience recurrent episodes of hypoxia, hypercapnia, or cardiovascular instability. The underlying cause of cardiopulmonary failure must be recognized and treated. No matter what the original etiology, if periods of hypoxia and hypotension go unrecognized and untreated, a fatal outcome is almost certain. In addition to the real danger of repeat cardiopulmonary arrest, there is a danger of secondary organ failure. The goal of postresuscitation support is to stabilize the patient to allow transportation to a facility where intensive care can be delivered.

The clinician should search for and treat the underlying cause of cardiopulmonary failure. Frequently, assessment of cardiopulmonary function is important. Monitoring for signs of inadequate pulmonary function, including shallow and uneven chest excursions, inadequate or unequal breath sounds, increased respiratory effort (eg, nasal flare, rib retraction), development of paradoxical ventilation (increased diaphragmatic efforts drawing chest wall in on inspiration), and, when possible, periodic ABG analysis, should be performed. Continuous ECG to monitor heart rate and rhythm can be informative. Repeat evaluation of peripheral circulation and end-organ perfusion by monitoring skin temperature, CRT, quality of distal pulses, mental status, and urine output is also important. Serial indirect blood pressure determinations can be useful.

Supportive measures, such as intranasal oxygen insufflation, maintaining body temperature with active warming, continuous intravenous glucose supplementation, and fluid therapy, are mandatory. Pressor and inotropic support should be given as needed. Dopamine, dobutamine, epinephrine, norepinephrine, and low-dose vasopressin are the most common useful choices. All these drugs must be given as continuous rate infusions with accurate intravenous infusion pumps through a central catheter. It should be remembered that the goal of pressor therapy is not to increase blood pressure but to increase and direct perfusion of tissues and maintain cardiac perfusion by maintaining diastolic pressure. As blood pressure increases, afterload increases and cardiac output drops. It is counterproductive to increase blood pressure at the expense of cardiac output. As blood pressure increases, more inotropic support of the heart is needed to support the cardiac output concurrently. For this reason, mixed α and β support (eg, dopamine, dobutamine, epinephrine) is useful [10].

Once perfusion and oxygen delivery are restored, it is vital to give glucose support to help clear metabolic acidosis. This is important because myocardial glycogen is generally depleted and supplementing glucose helps to prevent postasphyxia hypoglycemia. Glucose delivery should begin at a rate of 4 mg/kg/min. Monitoring blood glucose levels (every 30 minutes until stable) is necessary, because the glucose infusion rate frequently needs to be adjusted to prevent hyperglycemia or hypoglycemia. If tolerated, the glucose infusion rate should be increased to 8 mg/kg/min. Occasionally, the infusion rate needs to be greater than 8 mg/kg/min to satisfy glucose demands [29].

Birth resuscitation

Birth resuscitation is a special case of CPR requiring some modification in approach. Almost all newborns make the transition from fetal life without incident, but for those that do not, rapid recognition of the need to intervene is vital to achieve a successful outcome. Even when attending what is expected to be a normal birth, the clinician must monitor the progress of the foal's transition and be prepared to intervene when indicated.

The foals from high-risk pregnancy mares are at increased risk. Gravid dams are considered at high risk of a poor outcome of their gestation when they have a history of problems during past pregnancies or have developed a new problem during the current pregnancy. Problems in past gestations include placentitis, premature placental separation, recurrent dystocia, premature termination of pregnancy because of abortion or premature birth, prolonged pregnancies resulting in abnormal foals, and uterine artery hemorrhage. Current problems include precocious udder development; development of placentitis; discovery of twin pregnancy; detection of premature placental separation on ultrasound examination; overterm gestation relative to past gestations; musculoskeletal problems, such as fractures, laminitis, or lameness; development of endotoxemia, such as colic or colitis; development of hypotension or hypoxemia; recent abdominal surgical incision; development of a body wall hernia; neurologic disease marked by ataxia, weakness, or seizures; development of hydrops allantois or hydrops amnion; symptomatic pituitary hyperplasia; granulomatous intestinal disease; lymphosarcoma; melanomas in the pelvic canal; recent hemorrhage; and innumerable other problems. The list of possible problems leading to the risk of gestational problems is endless. Although it is useful to recognize the presence of these predisposing problems, when the mare's problem is viewed in terms of how it threatens fetal well-being, a clearer idea of the risk of an unsuccessful birth transition is possible. After understanding the threat, anticipation of problems at birth can lead to rational preparation and planning for birth resuscitation. Threats to fetal well-being include lack of placental perfusion; lack of oxygen delivery despite adequate perfusion; nutritional threats; placentitis or placental dysfunction; loss of fetal or maternal coordination of maturation; twin pregnancy; iatrogenic factors, such as drugs or other substances given to the mother; or early termination of pregnancy, such as induction or impending premature delivery. If any of these problems are evident, the foal is at high risk for having problems with the birth transition. Such cases should be enrolled in a high-risk pregnancy program, in which an attended hospital birth can decrease the risk of a poor outcome.

Initial assessment of the neonate should begin as the foal presents in the birth canal. A rapid evaluation of the peripheral pulse can be made when the vaginal positioning of the foal is checked. Relative pulse rate and strength form a basis for monitoring the expected changes during this dynamic period. Calculating an accurate pulse rate is unnecessary and counterproductive with the rapid changes occurring. The apical pulse can be assessed as soon as the chest clears the birth canal. Bradycardia (heart rate of 40 beats per minute [bpm] or less) is expected during forceful contractions while passing through the birth canal. A transient marked sinus arrhythmia commonly occurs when the first breaths are taken.

Once the chest clears the birth canal, the heart rate rapidly increases to 60 bpm or more. Persistent bradycardia with signs of poor perfusion is an indication for rapid intervention. Some foals maintain appropriate bradycardia with good perfusion. Calculating a modified Apgar score (Table 2) can help to determine the urgency and extent of intervention needed. The Apgar score is similar for all species, with the exception of the critical heart rate. This scoring system rates heart rate and rhythm (>60 bpm, regular rhythm = 2 points, irregular rhythm or <60 bpm = 1 point, absent rhythm = 0 points), respiratory rhythm (regular = 2 points, irregular = 1 point, absent = 0 point), body tone (sternal, active = 2 points; hypotonic = 1 point; atonic = 0 point) and response to stimuli (avoidance of stimulation = 2 points; grimace, weak response = 1 point; absent response = 0 point).

Table 2
Modified Apgar score (foal)

Score	2	1	0
Heart rate	>60 bpm, regular	<60 bpm, irregular	Absent
Respiratory rate	Regular	Irregular	Absent
Reflex nasal stimulation or ear tickle	Sneeze or cough, ear flick or head shake	Grimace, weak ear flick	No response
Muscle tone	Active sternal	Some flexion	Limp lateral

Score: 7–8, normal; 4–6, mild to moderate asphyxia (stimulate, provide intranasal oxygen, ventilate); 0–3, severe asphyxia (begin cardiopulmonary resuscitation).

Abbreviation: bpm, beats per minute.

Scores of 4 or less suggest the need for immediate intervention. Scores of 7 or 8 suggest that no intervention is needed. Scores of 5 or 6 suggest close observation, stimulation, and preparation for intervention. Although, traditionally, the Apgar score is recorded at 1, 5, and 10 minutes, if severe intrauterine stress has occurred, the need for resuscitation can be recognized before the 1-minute score is calculated when a nonperfusing cardiac rhythm is present.

An important step at birth is to clear the airway. The membranes should be removed from the nostrils as soon as the nose is visible. If meconium staining is present, the foal is depressed, and there is evidence of meconium "chunks," it is appropriate to suction the nasal passages and nasopharynx. If this is rewarding and the foal is severely asphyxiated, suctioning the trachea may be helpful. If the meconium is liquid (as with fetal diarrhea) or the foal is active and showing no evidence of significant depression, suctioning is contraindicated. Avoid overzealous suctioning because it can cause bradycardia and prolonged apnea. Because suctioning removes the air in the lungs, suctioning episodes should be limited to 10 to 15 seconds at a time with high flows of oxygen before and after each attempt. It is rare that a neonatal foal benefits from suctioning attempts, and suction itself is a high-risk procedure.

If spontaneous respiration and movement do not begin within seconds of birth, tactile stimulation is useful. Because the head usually presents first in a normal birth, tactile stimulation of the head (rubbing with a dry towel) is usually most rewarding. Rubbing the chest or stimulating the ear canal or nasal canal can also be rewarding. If spontaneous breathing efforts are not stimulated immediately in response to tactile stimulation, further efforts are unlikely to improve the situation. If apnea persists beyond 2 minutes, intubation and ventilation are indicated. Occasionally, the tactile stimulation caused by placing an intranasal oxygen cannula is sufficient stimulation to initiate breathing. This is also a good technique when breathing is present but is irregular with periodic apnea.

Apneic foals, who have an irregular and gasping respiratory pattern or remain bradycardic (<60 bpm), should receive respiratory support. If spontaneous respiratory efforts are present, give free-flow intranasal oxygen at a rate to 8 to 10 L/min. If no spontaneous respiration is present, intubate and ventilate. Use of oxygen during birth resuscitation has become controversial, and there is some evidence that room air is as effective and less harmful than 100% oxygen. It is likely that some oxygen enrichment is helpful, but 100% oxygen is not. Certainly, if oxygen is unavailable, room air is acceptable. If ventilatory equipment is unavailable, mouth-to-nose ventilation should be used.

With the first delivered breath, a prolonged inspiratory phase lasting approximately 5 seconds may help to ensure lung expansion. If perfusion is adequate but spontaneous ventilation is lacking, a delivered breath rate of 20 to 40 breaths per minute should be the goal. If there is a nonperfusing cardiac rhythm, ventilation should have a short inspiratory phase and low rate as during other forms of CPR. Consistent volumes of lung fluid should be seen escaping from the nostril during spontaneous and delivered ventilation.

If the asphyxia is mild and short lived, the heart rate should be greater than 60 bpm after 30 seconds of ventilation and should soon approach 100 bpm. Spontaneous respiratory efforts usually follow. Once they are present, the foal should be extubated and placed on free-flow intranasal oxygen. If the asphyxia is advanced and myocardial damage is present, bradycardia is likely to persist and cardiovascular support should be initiated. The more advanced the asphyxia is, the longer is the time until spontaneous ventilation occurs.

Chest compressions should be begun immediately if the foal remains bradycardic despite ventilation and develops a nonperfusing rhythm or if there is a nonperfusing rhythm or cardiac standstill at birth. If a perfusing spontaneous cardiac rhythm does not develop within 30 to 60 seconds of chest compressions, drug therapy should be initiated.

Thermal management is important in the compromised foal. Birthing areas of foals are usually cold. The healthy foal has little trouble handling cold environmental temperatures. The foal with even mild asphyxia can have difficulty with thermal control, however. Such a foal should be towel dried, placed on dry bedding, and provided an external heat source (eg, heat lamp, hot-water bottles, warm-water heating pads, or hot-air blanket). If the foal is depressed and remains hypothermic, moving it to a warm environment may be necessary.

As in all cases of cardiopulmonary failure, epinephrine should be given early and often. Epinephrine is the most useful drug for the treatment of cardiac failure secondary to birth asphyxia. The guidelines given for CPR should be used, with some exceptions. Atropine should not be used to treat early bradycardia in newborns. The initial bradycardia stimulated by hypoxia is vagally mediated. The atropine-mediated reversal of early hypoxic bradycardia is purely symptomatic, however, and does not treat the underlying cause (hypoxia). If the heart rate increases and the hypoxia is not corrected, the myocardium goes further into oxygen debt. This leads to an atropine-nonresponsive bradycardia caused by hypoxic myocardial damage. Treating the underlying cause, hypoxia, through ventilation with oxygen, chest compressions, and epinephrine reverses the bradycardia as rapidly as atropine therapy and prevents further damage. If the bradycardia does not respond despite effective CPR, atropine can then be considered.

Fluid therapy during the resuscitation of the newborn foal should be administered conservatively. The newborn is not volume depleted unless bleeding has occurred (eg, cord hemorrhage, fractured rib). Severe intrauterine distress results in a larger than normal extracellular fluid volume, and the neonate is born fluid overloaded, despite hypovolemia [29]. Fluid overloading can exacerbate a failing heart. High fluid rates can decrease coronary perfusion. Foals in hemorrhagic shock benefit from a bolus of non–glucose-containing fluids at a rate of 20 mL/kg if initial resuscitation attempts are not successful. Once spontaneous circulation is established and the foal is adequately oxygenated, treatment with glucose-containing fluids is indicated.

Despite successful return of spontaneous circulation, some foals retain the fetal circulation pattern, with pulmonary hypertension and right-to-left shunting through the foramen ovale and patent ductus arteriosus. These foals may benefit from ventilation with 100% oxygen, maintaining an arterial blood pH greater than 7.45 (do not allow the $Paco_2$ to decrease less than 30 mm Hg), or bicarbonate administration to produce metabolic alkalosis. The most effective treatment for persistent pulmonary hypertension is inhalation therapy with nitrous oxide at a rate of 5 to 20 ppm. Nitrous oxide causes pulmonary vasodilatation without affecting systemic blood pressure. Limited clinical experience shows nitrous oxide to be effective in foals, even at low concentrations.

Dystocia is a life-threatening event for the mare and the foal. Ex utero intrapartum treatment (EXIT) is a technique designed to support a foal during dystocia [45]. Briefly, the technique consists of identifying the nose of the fetal foal in the birth canal, intubating blindly, and beginning ventilation to resuscitate the foal before birth. As with CPR, capnography allows an estimate of cardiac output and helps to monitor the foal's condition. Intratracheal epinephrine can be given to assist with resuscitation. When EXIT is used in situations in which general anesthesia is necessary to correct the dystocia, there is a decrease in placental blood flow leading to decreased transfer of anesthetic agents and other drugs from maternal circulation to the fetus. EXIT is only possible if the nares are palpable in the birth canal and intubation is successful, which excludes a percentage of dystocia cases. EXIT procedures provide the luxury of time to correct the dystocia, a means to assess fetal viability, and a means to rescue fetal foals during dystocia [45].

Summary

When a pulseless cardiac rhythm is identified in a foal, it is vital to intervene using a well-planned scheme. The first priority should be to begin cardiac compressions and ventilation. Drug therapy always includes epinephrine and vasopressin. The cardiac rhythm should be established as shockable (VF or pulseless VT) or nonshockable (PEA or asystole). The treatment scheme branches, depending on the rhythm identified with a defibrillation, epinephrine, or lidocaine path or a continued CPR, epinephrine, or possible atropine path. Once a perfusing rhythm is established, postarrest stabilization requires careful monitoring and intervention. Birth resuscitation requires special considerations.

References

[1] Anonymous. 2005 American Heart Association guidelines for cardiopulmonary resuscitation and emergency cardiovascular care, part 7.2: management of cardiac arrest. Circulation 2005;112(Suppl IV):IV-58–66.

[2] Anonymous. 2005 American Heart Association guidelines for cardiopulmonary resuscitation and emergency cardiovascular care, part 7.1: adjuncts for airway control and ventilation. Circulation 2005;112(Suppl IV):IV-51–7.

[3] Aufderheide TP. The problem with and benefit of ventilations: should our approach be the same in cardiac and respiratory arrest? Curr Opin Crit Care 2006;12:207–12.

[4] Yannopoulos D, Tang W, Ruossos C, et al. Reducing ventilation frequency during cardiopulmonary resuscitation in a porcine model of cardiac arrest. Respir Care 2005;50: 628–35.

[5] Andrekaa P, Frenneaux MP. Haemodynamics of cardiac arrest and resuscitation. Curr Opin Crit Care 2006;12:198–203.

[6] Anonymous. 2005 American Heart Association guidelines for cardiopulmonary resuscitation and emergency cardiovascular care, part 3: overview of CPR. Circulation 2005; 112(Suppl IV):IV-12–8.

[7] Neumar RW, Ward KR. Adult resuscitation. In: Marx JR, editor. Rosen's emergency medicine: concepts and clinical practice. 6th edition. St. Louis (MO): Mosby; 2006. p. 75–95.

[8] Connick M, Berg RA. Femoral venous pulsations during open-chest cardiac massage. Ann Emerg Med 1994;24:1176–9.

[9] Anonymous. 2005 American Heart Association guidelines for cardiopulmonary resuscitation and emergency cardiovascular care, part 7.4: monitoring and medications. Circulation 2005;112(Suppl IV):IV-78–83.

[10] Palmer JE. Foal cardiopulmonary resuscitation. In: Orsini JA, Divers TJ, editors. Manual of equine emergencies: treatment and procedures. 2nd edition. Philadelphia: W.B. Saunders Co; 2003. p. 581–614.

[11] Fiser DH. Intraosseous infusion. N Engl J Med 1990;322:1579–81.

[12] Banerjee S, Singhi SC, Singh S, et al. The intraosseous route is a suitable alternative to intravenous route for fluid resuscitation in severely dehydrated children. Indian Pediatr 1994;31: 1511–20.

[13] Guy J, Haley K, Zuspan SJ. Use of intraosseous infusion in the pediatric trauma patient. J Pediatr Surg 1993;28:158–61.

[14] Berg RA. Emergency infusion of catecholamines into bone marrow. Am J Dis Child 1984; 138:810–1.

[15] Michael JR, Guerci AD, Koehler RC, et al. Mechanisms by which epinephrine augments cerebral and myocardial perfusion during cardiopulmonary resuscitation in dogs. Circulation 1984;69:822–35.

[16] Ditchey RV, Lindenfeld J. Failure of epinephrine to improve the balance between myocardial oxygen supply and demand during closed-chest resuscitation in dogs. Circulation 1988; 78:382–9.

[17] Tang W, Weil MH, Sun S, et al. Epinephrine increases the severity of postresuscitation myocardial dysfunction. Circulation 1995;92:3089–93.
[18] Rivers EP, Wortsman J, Rady MY, et al. The effect of the total cumulative epinephrine dose administered during human CPR on hemodynamic, oxygen transport, and utilization variables in the postresuscitation period. Chest 1994;106:1499–507.
[19] Lindner KH, Ahnefeld FW, Prengel AW. Comparison of standard and high-dose adrenaline in the resuscitation of asystole and electromechanical dissociation. Acta Anaesthesiol Scand 1991;35:253–6.
[20] Wenzel V, Krismer AC, Arntz HR, et al. A comparison of vasopressin and epinephrine for out-of-hospital cardiopulmonary resuscitation. N Engl J Med 2004;350:105–13.
[21] Guyette FX, Guimond GE, Hostler D, et al. Vasopressin administered with epinephrine is associated with a return of a pulse in out-of-hospital cardiac arrest. Resuscitation 2004;63: 277–82.
[22] Dauchot P, Gravenstein JS. Effects of atropine on the ECG in different age groups. Clin Pharmacol Ther 1971;12:272–80.
[23] Bernheim A, Fatio R, Kiowski W, et al. Atropine often results in complete atrioventricular block or sinus arrest after cardiac transplantation: an unpredictable and dose-independent phenomenon. Transplantation 2004;77:1181–5.
[24] Borer JS, Harrison LA, Kent KM, et al. Beneficial effect of lidocaine on ventricular electrical stability and spontaneous ventricular fibrillation during experimental myocardial infarction. Am J Cardiol 1976;37:860–3.
[25] Spear JF, Moore EN, Gerstenblith G. Effect of lidocaine on the ventricular fibrillation threshold in the dog during acute ischemia and premature ventricular contractions. Circulation 1972;46:65–73.
[26] Lie KI, Wellens HJ, van Capelle FJ, et al. Lidocaine in the prevention of primary ventricular fibrillation: a double-blind, randomized study of 212 consecutive patients. N Engl J Med 1974;291:1324–6.
[27] Anonymous. 2005 American Heart Association guidelines for cardiopulmonary resuscitation and emergency cardiovascular care, part 7.3: management of symptomatic bradycardia and tachycardia. Circulation 2005;112(Suppl IV) IV-67–IV-77.
[28] Anonymous. 2005 American Heart Association guidelines for cardiopulmonary resuscitation and emergency cardiovascular care, part 12: pediatric advanced life support. Circulation 2005;112(Suppl IV):IV-167–87.
[29] Palmer JE. Fluid therapy in the neonate—not your mother's fluid space! Vet Clin North Am Equine Pract 2004;20(1):63–75.
[30] Ditchey RV, Lindenfeld J. Potential adverse effects of volume loading on perfusion of vital organs during closed-chest resuscitation. Circulation 1984;69:181–9.
[31] Gentile NT, Martin GB, Appleton TJ, et al. Effects of arterial and venous volume infusion on coronary perfusion pressures during canine CPR. Resuscitation 1991;22:55–63.
[32] Kette F, Weil MH, Gazmuri RJ. Buffer solutions may compromise cardiac resuscitation by reducing coronary perfusion pressure. JAMA 1991;266:2121–6.
[33] Graf H, Leach W, Arieff AI. Evidence for a detrimental effect of bicarbonate therapy in hypoxic lactic acidosis. Science 1985;227:754–6.
[34] Stueven HA, Thompson B, Aprahamian C, et al. The effectiveness of calcium chloride in refractory electromechanical dissociation. Ann Emerg Med 1985;14:626–9.
[35] Stueven H, Thompson BM, Aprahamian C, et al. Use of calcium in prehospital cardiac arrest. Ann Emerg Med 1983;12:136–9.
[36] Ramoska EA, Spiller HA, Winter M, et al. A one-year evaluation of calcium channel blocker overdoses: toxicity and treatment. Ann Emerg Med 1993;22:196–200.
[37] Urban P, Scheidegger D, Buchmann B, et al. Cardiac arrest and blood ionized calcium levels. Ann Intern Med 1988;109:110–3.
[38] Cardenas-Rivero N, Chernow B, Stoiko MA, et al. Hypocalcemia in critically ill children. J Pediatr 1989;114:946–51.

[39] Broner CW, Stidham GL, Westenkirchner DF, et al. A prospective, randomized, double-blind comparison of calcium chloride and calcium gluconate therapies for hypocalcemia in critically ill children. J Pediatr 1990;117:986–9.

[40] Anonymous. 2005 American Heart Association guidelines for cardiopulmonary resuscitation and emergency cardiovascular care, part 5: electrical therapies. Circulation 2005; 112(Suppl IV):IV-35–46.

[41] Berg RA, Chapman FW, Berg MD, et al. Attenuated adult biphasic shocks compared with weight-based monophasic shocks in a swine model of prolonged pediatric ventricular fibrillation. Resuscitation 2004;61:189–97.

[42] van Alem AP, Chapman FW, Lank P, et al. A prospective, randomized and blinded comparison of first shock success of monophasic and biphasic waveforms in out-of-hospital cardiac arrest. Resuscitation 2003;58:17–24.

[43] Clark CB, Zhang Y, Davies LR, et al. Pediatric transthoracic defibrillation: biphasic versus monophasic waveforms in an experimental model. Resuscitation 2001;51:159–63.

[44] Gutgesell HP, Tacker WA, Geddes LA, et al. Energy dose for ventricular defibrillation of children. Pediatrics 1976;58:898–901.

[45] Palmer JE, Wilkins PA. How to use EXIT (ex-utero intrapartum treatment) to rescue foals during dystocia. In: Brokken TD, White SL, editors. Proceedings of 51st Annual Convention of the American Association of Equine Practitioners. Lexington (KY): American Association of Equine Practitioners; 2005. p. 281–3.

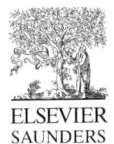

Index

Note: Page numbers of article titles are in **boldface** type.

A

N-Acetylcysteine, in oxidative stress management, 148–149

Activated charcoal, in poisoning management, 33–34

Airway(s), establishment of, in cardiopulmonary resuscitation in neonatal foals, 161–162

Airway disease, oxidative stress and, 137–140

Allopurinol, in oxidative stress management, 149

Analgesia/analgesics, in field fracture management, 116–117

Antibiotics. See *Antimicrobial agents*.

Anti-inflammatory drugs
    in envenomation management, 41
    in field fracture management, 117
    in synovial structure injury management, 106

Antimicrobial agents
    in envenomation management, 41
    in field fracture management, 117–118
    in synovial structure injury management, 106
    intra-articular, in synovial structure injury management, 106–108
    intrathecal, in synovial structure injury management, 106–108

Antimicrobial-impregnated PMMA, in synovial structure injury management, 108–109

Antioxidant(s)
    in oxidative stress management, 145–151
    in prevention of secondary injury to spinal cord, 93

Antivenin therapy, in envenomation management, 39–41

Apoptosis, SCI and, 84

Arachidonic acid metabolism, modulation of, in prevention of secondary injury to spinal cord, 94

Arthritis, septic, synovial structure injury and, 112

Arthroscopy, in synovial structure injury management, 110

Arthrotomy, in synovial structure injury management, 111

Atropine, in cardiopulmonary resuscitation in neonatal foals, 168–169

Axillary lacerations, 65–67

B

BALF. See *Bronchoalveolar lavage fluid (BALF)*.

Birth resuscitation, in neonatal foals, 173–177

Bismuth compounds, in poisoning management, 34

Blindness, acute, 61–62

Blunt chest trauma, 76

Body temperature, control of, in poisoning management, 32

Bronchoalveolar lavage fluid (BALF), 138

Bursa(ae), septic, synovial structure injury and, 112–113

C

Calcium, in cardiopulmonary resuscitation in neonatal foals, 170–171

Cardiac arrest, management of, in cardiopulmonary resuscitation in neonatal foals, 282

Cardiac compressions, in cardiopulmonary resuscitation in neonatal foals, 163–164

Cardiac output, effectiveness of, methods for measuring, in cardiopulmonary resuscitation in neonatal foals, 164–165

Cardiopulmonary failure, in neonatal foals, causes of, 158–161

Carolina rinse, in oxidative stress management, 150–151

Cathartic(s)
  oily, in poisoning management, 35
  saline, in poisoning management, 34–35

Central nervous system (CNS) support, in poisoning management, 31–32

Cerebrospinal fluid (CSF) analysis, in SCI diagnosis, 88

Charcoal, activated, in poisoning management, 33–34

Chest, flail, 68–70

Chest trauma, blunt, 76

Chest wounds, penetrating, 67–68

Circulation, trauma effects on, 90

Compression(s), cardiac, in cardiopulmonary resuscitation in neonatal foals, 163–164

Corneal laceration, 55–58

Corneal ulceration, 58–61

Corticosteroid(s)
  in envenomation management, 41–42
  in prevention of secondary injury to spinal cord, 91–92

Cushing's disease, equine, oxidative stress and, 144–145

D

Decontamination
  gastrointestinal, in poisoning management, 33–35
  skin, in poisoning management, 32–33

Defibrillation, electrical, in cardiopulmonary resuscitation in neonatal foals, 171–172

Diaphragmatic hernia, 74–75

Dimethyl sulfoxide (DMSO), in oxidative stress management, 149–150

Direct toxin removal, in poisoning management, 37–38

DMSO. See *Dimethyl sulfoxide (DMSO)*.

Drug(s), in cardiopulmonary resuscitation in neonatal foals, 167–171

E

Electrical defibrillation, in cardiopulmonary resuscitation in neonatal foals, 171–172

Elimination, increase in, in poisoning management, 36

Endoscopy, in synovial structure injury management, 110

Envenomation. See also *Poisoning*.
  management of, **38–42**
    antibiotics in, 41
    anti-inflammatory drugs in, 41
    antivenin therapy in, 39–41
    corticosteroids in, 41–42
    principles in, 1042
    stabilization of acutely ill patient in, 39
    tetanus toxoid in, 41

Enzymatic conversion, in poisoning management, 36

Epinephrine, in cardiopulmonary resuscitation in neonatal foals, 167

Equine Cushing's disease, oxidative stress and, 144–145

Equine motor neuron disease, oxidative stress and, 142–143

Equine pituitary pars intermedia dysfunction, oxidative stress and, 144–145

Erythropoietin, in prevention of secondary injury to spinal cord, 95

Excretion, promotion of, in poisoning management, 36–37

Exercise, oxidative stress and, 140–142

Eyelid lacerations, 54–55

F

Field fractures
  assessment of
    general principles of, 119–120
    radiography in, 119–120
  management of, **115–131**, 120
    analgesia in, 116–117
    antibiotics in, 117–118
    anti-inflammatory drugs in, 117
    fluid therapy in, 118–119

medical stabilization in
general principles of,
115–119
patient assessment in,
115–116
sedation in, 116–117
tetanus prophylaxis in, 117–118
thrombosis prevention in, 119
of appendicular skeleton, 120–127
distal limb, 122–123
distal metacarpal or metatarsal
condyle, 123–124
fracture stabilization, principles
of, 120–122
humerus or femur and above this
level, 126–127
mid- and proximal radius,
124–125
midforelimb or middle hind limb,
124
olecranon, 124
tibia, 125–126
of skull, mandible, and maxilla,
127–129
prognosis of, 120
transportation of equine patients with,
129

Fire and smoke inhalation injury, **17–28**.
See also *Fire injuries; Inhalation
injuries*.
clinical signs of, 21–23
diagnosis of, 24–25
first response and disaster
preparedness for, 18–19
prognosis of, 25–27
treatment of, goals in, 25–27

Fire injuries, pathophysiology of, 19–20

First response and disaster preparedness,
for fire and smoke inhalation injury,
18–19

Fistula(ae)
rib, 71–72
sternal, 71–72

Flail chest, 68–70

Flood(s)
causes of, 1
planning for, 1–6
prevalence of, 1
response to, 6–8

Flood injury, in horses, **1–17**
gastrointestinal dysfunction, 12–14
handling and restraint after, 9
hoof problems, 11
integument and musculoskeletal
injuries, 9–11

neurologic disease, 14–15
ophthalmic injuries, 11–12
prevention of, 1–6
respiratory disease, 15–16
response to, 6–8
triage and medical treatment for, 8–9

Fluid(s)
in cardiopulmonary resuscitation in
neonatal foals, 169–170
in field fracture management, 118–119

Foal(s), neonatal. See also *Neonatal foals.*
resuscitation in, **157–180**. See also
Resuscitation, in neonatal foals.

Fracture(s)
field. See *Field fractures.*
frontal, 128–129
mandible, 127–129
maxilla, 127–129
nasal, 128–129
orbital, 52–54
premaxillary, 127–128
rib, 70–71
skull, 127–129

Free radical(s), trauma effects on, 82

Free radical scavengers, in prevention of
secondary injury to spinal cord, 93

G

Ganglioside(s), in prevention of secondary
injury to spinal cord, 92–93

Gastric lavage, in poisoning management,
33

Gastrointestinal decontamination, in
poisoning management, 33–35

Gastrointestinal dysfunction, flood-related,
12–14

Glutathione redox ratio (GRR), 138

GRR. See *Glutathione redox ratio (GRR).*

H

Hernia(s), diaphragmatic, 74–75

Hoof problems, flood-related, 11

I

Immunologic response, SCI and, 83–84

Immunosuppressive therapy, in prevention
of secondary injury to spinal cord, 95

Inflammatory response, SCI and, 83–84

Inhalation injuries, pathophysiology of, 20–21

Integument injuries, flood-related, 9–11

International Standards Organization/ American National Standards Institute (ISO/ANSI), 3

Intra-articular antimicrobial therapy, in synovial structure injury management, 106–108

Intrathecal antimicrobial agents, in synovial structure injury management, 106–108

Ion homeostasis dysregulation, SCI and, 83

Ischemia-reperfusion injury, oxidative stress and, 134–137

ISO/ANSI. See *International Standards Organization/American National Standards Institute (ISO/ANSI)*.

J

Joint disease, oxidative stress and, 143–144

K

Kaolin-pectin, in poisoning management, 34

Keratitis, ulcerative, 58–61

L

Laceration(s)
 axillary, 65–67
 corneal, 55–58
 eyelid, 54–55
 pectoral, 65–67

Lidocaine, in cardiopulmonary resuscitation in neonatal foals, 169

Lipid peroxidation, trauma and, 82

M

Magnesium, in cardiopulmonary resuscitation in neonatal foals, 169

Mandible, fractures of, 127–129

Mandibular and premaxillary fractures, 127–128

Maxilla, fractures of, 127–129

Metabolism, arachidonic acid, in prevention of secondary injury to spinal cord, 94

Mineral(s), supplementation with, in oxidative stress management, 148

Minocycline, in prevention of secondary injury to spinal cord, 94

Musculoskeletal injuries, flood-related, 9–11

N

Nasal, frontal, and maxillary bone fractures, 128–129

Necrosis(es), SCI and, 84

Neonatal foals
 cardiopulmonary failure in, causes of, 158–161
 resuscitation in, **157–180**. See also *Resuscitation, in neonatal foals*.

Neurologic disease, flood-related, 14–15

O

Oily cathartics, in poisoning management, 35

Ophthalmic emergencies, **47–63**
 acute blindness, 61–62
 corneal ulceration, 58–61
 orbital trauma, 47–58
 ulcerative keratitis, 58–61

Ophthalmic injuries, flood-related, 11–12

Opioid receptor antagonists, in prevention of secondary injury to spinal cord, 92

Orbital fractures, 52–54

Orbital trauma, 47–58
 corneal laceration, 55–58
 eyelid lacerations, 54–55
 initial evaluation in, 47–48
 ocular examination in, 48–52
 orbital fractures, 52–54

Oxidative stress, **133–155**
 airway disease and, 137–140
 conditions associated with, 134–145
 defined, 133
 described, 133–134
 equine Cushing's disease and, 144–145
 equine motor neuron disease and, 142–143
 equine pituitary pars intermedia dysfunction and, 144–145
 exercise and, 140–142
 ischemia-reperfusion injury and, 134–137
 joint disease and, 143–144
 treatment for
  N-acetylcysteine in, 148–149
  allopurinol in, 149
  Carolina rinse in, 150–151
  DMSO in, 149–150

future antioxidant therapies in, 151
multiple vitamin or mineral supplementation in, 148
therapeutic antioxidants in, 145–151
21-aminosteroids in, 150
U-74389G in, 150
vitamin C in, 146–147
vitamin E and selenium in, 145–146

P

Pectoral lacerations, 65–67

PELF. See *Pulmonary epithelial lining fluid (PELF)*.

Penetrating chest wounds, 67–68

PMMA. See *Polymethylmethacrylate (PMMA)*.

Pneumomediastinum, 73

Pneumothorax, 72–73

Poisoning. See also *Envenomation*.
management of, **29–45**
activated charcoal in, 33–34
bismuth compounds in, 34
body temperature control in, 32
cardiovascular function maintenance in, 30–31
CNS support in, 31–32
direct toxin removal in, 37–38
enzymatic conversion in, 36
excretion promotion in, 36–37
gastric lavage in, 33
gastrointestinal decontamination in, 33–35
increasing elimination in, 36
kaolin-pectin in, 34
oily cathartics in, 35
prevention of further exposure in, 29–30
principles in, 29–38
respiration maintenance in, 30
saline cathartics in, 34–35
skin decontamination in, 32–33
stabilization of acutely ill patient, 30–32
topical exposure–related, 32–33
whole-bowel irrigation in, 35

Polymethylmethacrylate (PMMA), antimicrobial-impregnated, in synovial structure injury management, 108–109

Pulmonary epithelial lining fluid (PELF), 138

R

Radiography, in field fracture assessment, 119–120

Regional limb perfusion, in synovial structure injury management, 108

Respiratory disease, flood-related, 15–16

Resuscitation
birth, in neonatal foals, 173–177
in neonatal foals, **157–180**
atropine in, 168–169
birth resuscitation, 173–177
calcium in, 170–171
cardiac arrest management in, 282
cardiac compressions in, 163–164
clinical approach to, 161–177
drug therapy in, 167–171
electrical defibrillation in, 171–172
epinephrine in, 167
establishing airway in, 161–162
fluids in, 169–170
lidocaine in, 169
magnesium in, 169
measuring cardiac output effectiveness in, methods for, 164–165
postresuscitation support, 172–173
sodium bicarbonate in, 170
vascular access in, 165–166
vasopressin in, 168
ventilation in, 162–163

Rib(s)
fistulae of, 71–72
fractures of, 70–71

S

Saline cathartics, in poisoning management, 34–35

SCI. See *Spinal cord injury (SCI)*.

Sedation, in field fracture management, 116–117

Septic arthritis, synovial structure injury and, 112

Septic bursae, synovial structure injury and, 112–113

Septic tenosynovitis, synovial structure injury and, 112

Skin decontamination, in poisoning management, 32–33

Skull, fractures of, 127–129

Smoke inhalation injury, **17–28**. See also *Fire and smoke inhalation injury*.

Sodium bicarbonate, in cardiopulmonary resuscitation in neonatal foals, 170

Sodium channel blockers, in prevention of secondary injury to spinal cord, 93–94

SPAOPD. See *Summer pasture-associated obstructive pulmonary diseases (SPAOPD)*.

Spinal cord injury (SCI)
  apoptosis and, 84
  cervicothoracic, 86–87
  clinical signs of, 84–88
  diagnosis of, 84–88
    CSF analysis in, 88
    neuroimaging in, 88
  excitotoxicity and, 82–83
  free radicals and lipid peroxidation, 82–83
  high cervical, 86
  inflammatory and immunologic response to, 83–84
  ion homeostasis dysregulation and, 83
  lumbosacral, 87
  management of, 89–95
    acute, 89–90
    in prevention of secondary injury, 91–95
      antioxidants, 93
      corticosteroids, 91–92
      erythropoietin, 95
      free radical scavengers, 93
      gangliosides, 92–93
      immunosuppressive therapy, 95
      minocycline, 94
      modulation of arachidonic acid metabolism, 94
      opioid receptor antagonists, 92
      sodium channel blockers, 93–94
      TRH, 93
      TRH analogues, 93
  necrosis and, 84
  pathophysiology of, 79–84
  sacrococcygeal, 87–88
  thoracolumbar, 87
  vascular abnormalities due to, 81–82

Sternum, fistulae of, 71–72

Stress, oxidative, **133–155**. See also *Oxidative stress*.

Summer pasture-associated obstructive pulmonary diseases (SPAOPD), 140

Synovial structures, injury to, **101–114**
  diagnosis of, 102–104
    modalities in, 103–104
    patient history in, 102–103
    physical examination in, 102–103
    wound preparation in, 103
  pathogenesis of, 101–102
  prognosis for, 111–113
  septic arthritis due to, 112
  septic bursae due to, 112–113
  septic tenosynovitis due to, 112
  treatment of, 104–111
    antimicrobial-impregnated PMMA in, 108–109
    arthroscopy in, 110
    arthrotomy in, 111
    endoscopy in, 110
    intra-articular or intrathecal antimicrobial therapy in, 106–108
    plan for, 104–106
    regional limb perfusion in, 108
    synovial lavage and drainage in, 110–111
    systemic antimicrobial and anti-inflammatory therapy in, 106
    through-and-through lavage in, 110–111
    ventral drainage in, 111

T

Temperature, body, control of, in poisoning management, 32

Tenosynovitis, septic, synovial structure injury and, 112

Tetanus, vaccination for, in field fracture management, 117–118

Tetanus toxoid, in envenomation management, 41

Thoracic trauma, **65–78**
  axillary lacerations, 65–67
  blunt chest trauma, 76
  diaphragmatic hernia, 74–75
  flail chest, 68–70
  pectoral lacerations, 65–67
  penetrating chest wounds, 67–68
  pneumomediastinum, 73
  pneumothorax, 72–73
  rib fistulae, 71–72
  rib fractures, 70–71
  sternal fistulae, 71–72

Thrombosis(es), prevention of, in field fracture management, 119

Thyrotropin-releasing hormone (TRH), in prevention of secondary injury to spinal cord, 93

Thyrotropin-releasing hormone (TRH) analogues, in prevention of secondary injury to spinal cord, 93

Trauma
   chest, blunt, 76
   neurologic sequelae of, **79–99.** See also *Spinal cord injury (SCI).*
      airway management for, 90
      circulation-related, 90
      clinical signs of, 84–88
      diagnosis of, 84–88
      excitotoxicity and, 82–83
      free radicals and lipid peroxidation and, 82
      management of, acute, 89–90
   orbital, 47–58. See also *Orbital trauma.*
   thoracic, **65–78.** See also *Thoracic trauma.*
   vascular abnormalities due to, 81–82

TRH analogues. See *Thyrotropine-releasing hormone (TRH) analogues.*

Trough-and-through lavage, in synovial structure injury management, 110–111

21-Aminosteroids, in oxidative stress management, 150

U

U-74389G, in oxidative stress management, 150

Ulceration, corneal, 58–61

Ulcerative keratitis, 58–61

US Department of Agriculture (USDA) National Animal Identification System, 3

US Horse Industry Equine Species Working Group, 3

V

Vascular abnormalities, SCI and, 81–82

Vascular access, in cardiopulmonary resuscitation in neonatal foals, 165–166

Vasopressin, in cardiopulmonary resuscitation in neonatal foals, 168

Ventilation, in cardiopulmonary resuscitation in neonatal foals, 162–163

Ventral drainage, in synovial structure injury management, 111

Vitamin(s)
   C, in oxidative stress management, 146–147
   E, selenium and, in oxidative stress management, 145–146
   supplementation with, in oxidative stress management, 148

W

Whole-bowel irrigation, in poisoning management, 35

Wound(s). See also specific types, e.g., *Laceration(s).*
   chest, penetrating, 67–68

Moving?

Make sure your subscription moves with you!

To notify us of your new address, find your **Clinics Account Number** (located on your mailing label above your name), and contact customer service at:

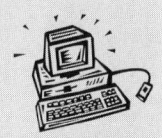

E-mail: elspcs@elsevier.com

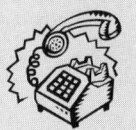

800-654-2452 (subscribers in the U.S. & Canada)
407-345-4000 (subscribers outside of the U.S. & Canada)

Fax number: 407-363-9661

Elsevier Periodicals Customer Service
6277 Sea Harbor Drive
Orlando, FL 32887-4800

*To ensure uninterrupted delivery of your subscription, please notify us at least 4 weeks in advance of move.

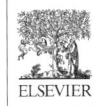